Lewis Russell qualified as a state registered chiropodist at the London Foot Hospital in 1966. He then worked at the Greenwich District Hospital and as an assistant in a private practice in Sidcup, Kent. He also started teaching chiropody part-time at the London Foot Hospital, becoming full-time there in 1969. He took up a new teaching post at the Chelsea School of Chiropody in 1972. Eight years later he moved to Plymouth as deputy head of the newly opened School of Chiropody, becoming head in 1986.

Lewis Russell is married with two children. His wife is also a state registered chiropodist and teacher.

Bob Hardy joined Clarks Shoes Ltd as a Technical Student after leaving school. He then worked in the company's manufacturing and development areas. He is now Fitting Services Manager, and is responsible for retail staff training and representing Clarks Shoes on the Foot Health Council and the Children's Foot Health Register. He is also a member of the Society of Shoefitters.

Bob Hardy was born and still lives in Street, Somerset. He is married with two children.

HEALTHY FEET

LEWIS RUSSELL FChS, SRCh AND BOB HARDY MSSF

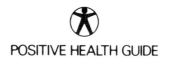

POSITIVE HEALTH GUIDE

© Bob Hardy and Lewis Russell 1988

© Illustrations and photographs on pages 18,
19, 20, 21, 22, 23, 24, 59, 91, and 97 are the subject
of copyright and are reproduced with the kind
permission of the copyright owner C. & J. Clark
International Limited of Street, Somerset, England

First published in 1988 by
Macdonald Optima, a division of
Macdonald & Co. (Publishers) Ltd

A member of Maxwell Pergamon Publishing Corporation plc

British Library Cataloguing in Publication Data

Russell, Lewis
    Healthy feet.
    1. Man. Feet. Care
    I. Title   II. Hardy, Bob
    617'.585

    ISBN 0-356-15190-5

Macdonald & Co. (Publishers) Ltd
3rd Floor
Greater London House
Hampstead Road
London NW1 7QX

Photoset in 11pt Times by   Tek Art Limited, Croydon, Surrey

Printed and bound in Great Britain at the University Press, Cambridge

CONTENTS

ACKNOWLEDGMENTS

We would like to thank Brenda Correa, Pamela Mogg and Tracy Walton for typing the manuscripts. Thanks also to the Children's Foot Health Register, the Society of Shoe Fitters, the Disabled Living Foundation and the British Footwear Manufacturers' Federation for allowing information about them to be published, and to Clarks Shoes Limited for granting permission to use various slides and pictures plus information from their Foot Health Programme.

The publishers would like to thank Maggie Raynor for the line drawings and Zefa of London for the cover photograph.

1

ANATOMY AND PHYSIOLOGY OF THE FOOT

The foot is a highly complex and intricate structure whose care and well-being are usually ignored until it is unable to perform the normal functions we expect of it.

Although the foot can seldom be considered in isolation, being only one small part of the human locomotor system, it does, perhaps more than any other structure or part of the body, have to contend with abuse and misuse from its owner. Most feet start life as perfectly-shaped attractive structures, but by middle age they have been turned by their owners into distorted and poorly-functioning objects which they hide away in their footwear.

The variety of odd shapes that feet develop over the years has much to do with the very large number of individual bones and joints found in our feet. It is extraordinary that in such a small area there are 28 bones (including the two tiny sesamoid bones) in each foot. Compare that to the number of bones between your hip and ankle – a mere four, including the knee-cap.

So let us start off this book by looking at the structure and workings of the feet.

BONES

Bones provide a framework and the supporting structure for many of the body's tissues.

Bone is a living structure, its cells are constantly remodelling and, when necessary, repairing themselves during the course of a lifetime. A cross section through bone reveals a hard, tough outer shell with an open meshwork or hollow section inside, which produces a strong, firm, but light structure. The marrow inside some of the bones is very important as it produces the red blood cells which carry vital substances around our blood vessels.

When part of a bone comes into contact with another bone, the two are said to 'articulate' if movement occurs between them. To help in this movement, and to save the bones from grating on each other, the ends of the bones are covered with cartilage which is a softer and smoother substance. The bones are held together by ligaments (see page 5), which help to stop unwanted movement, and, with other tissues, form a capsule around the two ends of bone to produce a joint.

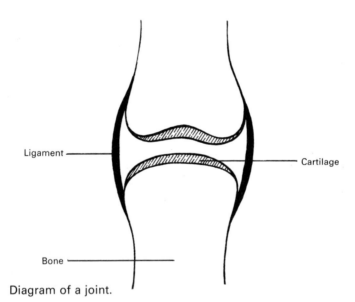

Diagram of a joint.

Joints have a delicate lining called a synovial membrane which produces a lubricating fluid inside the joint called synovial fluid. This substance is important in helping to reduce the wear and tear on the surfaces inside the joint, especially the cartilage.

The amount and type of movement which is possible in a joint will depend both on the shape of the joint surfaces of the two bones and the structures which hold the bones together – the ligaments, muscles and tendons. If the joint is a ball and socket type, e.g. the hip joint, then an enormous range of movement is possible, compared to the flat joints found between some of the small bones in the foot, e.g. the cuneiforms, where only small amounts of sliding movement are possible.

Bones in the foot

The foot is usually defined as starting from the ankle, so the two most important bones at the rear of the foot are the calcaneum (heel bone) and the talus which connects the heel

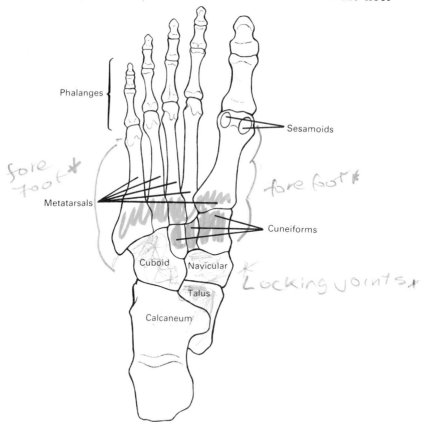

Bones of the foot – plantar (sole) surface. Medial (inner) border. Lateral (outer) border.

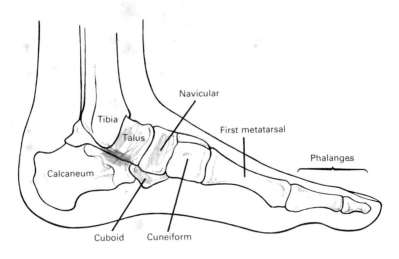

Bones of the foot – medial (inner) border.

to the leg. The talus sits on top of the calcaneum and the joint which is formed between the two bones is called the sub-taloid joint. This joint is very important in allowing certain movements known as pronation and supination (which will be explained on pages 11–12) to take place in the foot. The calcaneum projects backwards to form the heel and to provide a lever for the Achilles tendon.

In front of the talus is the boat-shaped bone called the navicular (from the Latin for small boat), while in front of the calcaneum is the cuboid (cube-shaped) bone. The joints formed by the calcaneum and talus with the cuboid and navicular are known collectively as the mid-tarsal joint. This joint allows the front part of the foot to turn inwards or outwards relative to the rear of the foot. It is important in the foot's function as it becomes locked during the phase in walking when the foot is bearing weight (see page 11). If the joint does not lock, the forefoot is unstable and damage can occur, leading to malformed toes and bunions.

In front of the navicular lie three small, wedge-shaped bones called the cuneiforms. The five metatarsals articulate with the cuneiforms and cuboid and comprise the first part of the forefoot. The metatarsals are the longest bones in the foot and articulate with the bones of the toes, which are called phalanges. The big toe is known as the hallux, and has two phalanges, whilst the four lesser toes have three phalanges each.

The joints between the metatarsals and the phalanges form the bending part of the forefoot, making them very important in normal walking. They are called the metatarso-phalangeal joints. In common with the toes, these joints are numbered by the chiropodist; the big toe (hallux) is the first toe, the middle toe is the third toe, and the little toe is the fifth toe. The first metatarso-phalangeal joint is therefore the big toe joint. Long bones such as a metatarsal are also described as having a base, shaft and head, and these are terms which will be used later in this book.

Under the first metatarso-phalangeal joint are usually found two very small bones known as sesamoids which are embedded in a tendon of a muscle. These tiny bones protect the joint by transmitting stress away, and also provide a pulley function for the important muscles which act on the big toe during walking.

LIGAMENTS

Ligament joins bone to bone and is composed of fibrous tissue which is strong yet has some elasticity. It can adapt to change, so that if it is put under tension it will extend in the course of time to become longer, whilst if it is allowed to become slack it will shorten to take up the slack. (This is known as Davis's law, and other tissues such as tendons and skin will also adapt in the same way.)

A common condition seen in the forefoot is the dislocation or partial dislocation (subluxation) of the toes. If a toe is buckled by the shoe and is held in that position for a long period the soft tissue around the joints will adapt by shortening or lengthening, eventually locking the toe in this fixed position. Unlike the sudden dislocation of a shoulder or elbow in a fall, the dislocation of a toe will take several years to develop and its correction is very difficult without surgery.

In contrast, if a ligament is suddenly stretched it is likely to tear or completely rupture, which usually causes considerable pain and immobility. This commonly occurs when the ankle is sprained, and is discussed on page 122.

5

MUSCLES

The muscles which send their tendons into the foot, plus the muscles which originate within it, are very numerous. The ability to use most of the smaller muscles within the foot are lost to most of us, although it is interesting that some severely handicapped people are able to develop fine movements of their toes so that they can work machinery or become artists.

Muscles if overused or deprived of oxygen (because of a poor blood supply) become painful and this can be seen in the leg and foot, especially in athletes and in some medical conditions. Tendons, which attach muscles to bones, can also become painful when damaged by stresses similar to those that cause torn ligaments – the large tendon at the heel, the Achilles tendon, is a common site for such problems.

The muscles at the back of the leg – the calf – are very important for their pumping action, which squeezes the blood in the veins back to the heart. This pumping occurs as the muscle contracts and relaxes, squeezing the veins around it, and allowing fresh blood from the lungs and heart to flow into the leg and foot. When this muscle pump fails, in conditions such as polio, the leg and foot become swollen and cold, causing problems with footwear and probably chilblains, unless advice is sought.

If high-heeled shoes are worn over a period of years, the muscle in the calf will respond by shortening. This means that returning to a flat-heeled shoe can be a painful procedure – the muscle and tendon should be allowed to adapt and lengthen gradually by reducing the heel height over a period of weeks.

THE ARCHES OF THE FOOT

Many people seem excessively concerned about the arches of the foot and the benefits of a high arch compared to that of a low one and vice versa.

The foot is arched from front to back (the longitudinal arch) and from side to side (the transverse arch). The longitudinal arch can be seen on the skeleton of a foot on both its inner border (the medial longitudinal arch) and also on its outer border (the lateral longitudinal arch). The inner arch is the higher and more flexible, and is used as a shock absorber during walking and running. The outer longitudinal arch is almost non-existent, lacks flexibility and is a supportive structure rather than a dynamic one.

The transverse arch runs from one side of the foot to the other and is highest on the inner border. It is seen clearly in the mid-part of the foot. Although some people still talk of an arch across the metatarsal heads (the metatarsal arch), it has been proved that this does not exist in the normal foot thus making the popular 'dropped metatarsal arch' condition a fallacy.

A wet footprint seen on a dry surface will usually show the parts of the foot – the heel, the outer border of the foot, the metatarsal head area and some of the toes – which come in contact with the ground and bear weight. The arch area on the inner border of the foot is usually seen to be the only non-weight-bearing area in the normal foot.

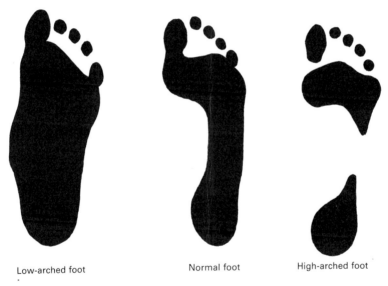

Low-arched foot   Normal foot   High-arched foot

Footprints showing different arch heights.

These arches are not dependent on the bones; in fact the shape of the bones plays only a small part in the structure of the arches. Instead the arches of the feet depend principally on the very strong ligaments and fascia found in the sole of the foot, and also the foot muscles which span from the heel to the forefoot plus the long muscle tendons which originate in the leg. The strength of the ligaments and fascia is such that they can control and support the arch during standing even when subjected to high loading, and it is only during walking and running that the muscles play a part in supporting the arch.

A foot with a low longitudinal arch is not necessarily a weak one providing that it can form an arch when the foot comes up on tiptoe. This simulates the movement of the foot during the propulsive phase in walking when the foot must be arched and rigid. The foot which is highly arched (pes cavus) and rigid all of the time, even on standing when it should be relaxed, is usually much more of a problem to its owner than the flexible low-arched foot. These foot types are discussed in more detail on pages 37–9.

BLOOD VESSELS

The blood vessels which carry blood away from the heart are the arteries, while those that take the blood back to the heart are the veins. The contractions of the heart produce enough pressure in the circulation system to pump the blood to the feet, but for its return journey to the heart it must rely on the squeezing action of the calf muscles mentioned just now and the one-way valves in the veins, which stop the blood from running back into the feet.

Many people are surprised that pulses can be felt in the foot, but the two arteries which can be felt there give the chiropodist or doctor an indication of the quality and quantity of the local blood supply. The artery which can be felt on the top of the foot is known as the dorsalis pedis artery whilst the other,

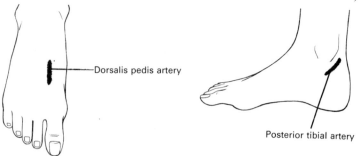

Dorsalis pedis artery

Posterior tibial artery

Pulses in the foot.

8

which is more difficult to feel, is found on the inside border of the heel below the ankle bone and is called the posterior tibial artery. The problems which can arise from poor circulation in the feet are dealt with in more detail in Chapter 6.

NERVES

The nerves within the feet are as sensitive as those in the hands, and are responsible for sending messages back to the brain regarding pain, touch, temperature and position. Problems with these sensory nerves in such conditions as diabetes can produce areas in the foot in which there is no sensation. As these areas are usually associated with areas of poor blood circulation, they require skilful attention in order to prevent skin damage and ulceration; if such damage does occur, it may not be initially noticed, due to the lack of sensation.

Not all nerves, however, are sensory. Many are responsible for the action of the muscles, and these motor nerves can become defective in conditions such as polio, multiple sclerosis and stroke, leaving the foot and leg paralysed.

SUBCUTANEOUS TISSUE

The depth of tissue between the skin and bone varies throughout the foot. Over the tops of the toes the tissue is very thin, while under the metatarso-phalangeal joints and under the heel the tissue will be very thick. This thick tissue on the sole of the foot is a useful buffer, protecting the bones and joints from damage during the trauma of walking and running.

As we age this layer of fatty padding tends to reduce, unlike fatty deposits elsewhere in the body. This means that often the foot of the elderly person is less well protected from pressure than a young person's, and this may lead to pain and discomfort or a higher tendency to form corns and callosities.

SKIN

The thickness of the skin varies in different parts of the body. On the sole of the foot, which is expected to bear considerable weight and undergo a great deal of stress, it is thicker than in most other parts of the body. Also, on the sole of the foot the skin is attached tightly to the tissues underneath, whereas on the tops of the toes it is loosely attached and can be easily lifted in a fold.

The skin is an important organ of the body because of its varied functions. It acts as a protective layer, preventing penetration by germs, fluids and damaging sunlight. It also acts as part of the body's mechanism to keep its temperature relatively constant and to rid itself of certain waste products. And the nerve endings within it make it capable of sensing hot, cold, pain and touch.

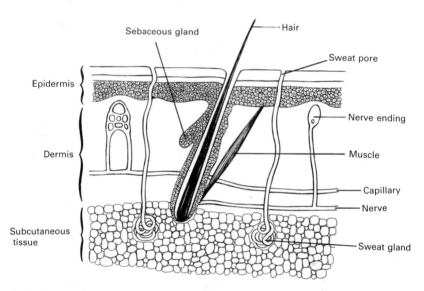

Structure of the skin.

The skin is divided into two main regions; the outer layer is known as the epidermis and the deeper layer is the dermis.

The epidermis
This is the most superficial part of the skin, and is itself divided into various layers. Its deepest layer is the most active, as it is the site of cell division. The cells produced in this layer then move upwards towards the skin's outer surface and as they do

so they change from living cells into dead cells containing a tough horny protein called keratin. This process of cells moving and changing composition is important as it produces the tough protective outer barrier we all need.

These dead cells are then shed from the skin's surface and are continuously replaced by new skin cells formed in the lower layer.

The dermis

This is the layer underneath the epidermis, which contains nerves, blood vessels, ducts from the sweat glands and the shafts of the hair follicles. It is the major portion of the skin and through it the epidermis obtains its nourishment and sensitivity.

HOW WE WALK

The process of walking and running is probably more complex than most people imagine. Let us have a look at this process in a little detail.

The foot first touches the ground on the outside of the heel. Weight is then transferred onto the foot's inner border and the forefoot touches the ground. At this point the foot is at its most mobile, with the long arch under the foot at its lowest. Most of the movement of the foot into this low-arched position takes place at the sub-taloid joint under the ankle, and the foot is said to be **pronated** when in this position. As the body's weight is transferred from the heel to the toes, the foot must change from this low-arched mobile flexible shape into a rigid lever.

After pronation, the load on the foot moves to the outer side of the foot which increases the height of the arch and produces a rigid foot which makes a better lever for the propulsion now required. This rigid state of the foot is known as **supination** and this movement also takes place mainly at the sub-taloid joint.

The foot, however, does not work in isolation, and movements of pronation or supination will be accompanied by movements of the leg, knee, hip and trunk. For example, when the foot pronates, the leg will rotate internally causing movements at the knee and hip; likewise, when the foot is supinating the leg must rotate externally, with corresponding movements at the knee and hip.

11

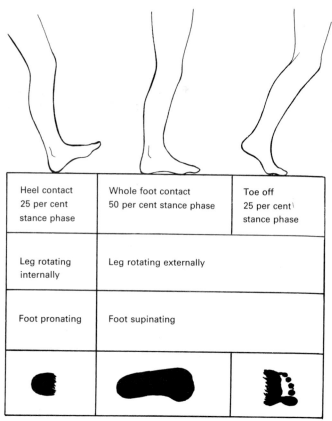

Heel contact 25 per cent stance phase	Whole foot contact 50 per cent stance phase	Toe off 25 per cent stance phase
Leg rotating internally	Leg rotating externally	
Foot pronating	Foot supinating	

The walking cycle.

And don't forget that while these movements are taking place in the foot that bears the body's weight, the opposite foot is swinging in the air, taking no weight but moving into position for the heel to strike the ground and begin its process of pronation and supination.

2

GENERAL FOOT CARE

A little care and attention plus common sense should provide us with trouble-free feet. Following the points outlined in this chapter – on footwear, hygiene, skin care, exercise, etc. – should also help.

FOOTWEAR

Shoes and hose (socks, stockings, tights, etc.) will have a direct effect on the welfare of the foot, so special care should be taken in their selection.

The proper shoe for the occasion should always be the most important consideration. For example, high-heeled court shoes are meant to be worn for short periods at social events, and not for walking around the supermarket or shopping in the sales.

The ideal shoe for both men and women is one that is adequate in length, width and depth, causing no pressure on the toes. It should have a heel no higher than 1½ inches (3–4 cm) and a lace, buckle or some other fastening which holds the shoe securely onto the foot. A shoe which can be slipped on and off the foot without undoing the fastening is not a proper fit. (The details of fittings and shoe properties are dealt with in greater detail in Chapters 7–10.)

Socks and tights can also have a restricting effect on the foot and toes if they are too short and are made of materials which stretch and therefore pull back on the toes. The most vulnerable wearer of such hosiery will be the young child, whose toes can be permanently buckled by the use of badly fitted socks or tights.

Ideally socks and shoes should be changed daily, the socks so that they can be washed and the shoes so that they can have a chance for the moisture absorbed into the leather from the person's sweat to evaporate and dry naturally.

HYGIENE AND SKIN CARE

The feet encased in shoes and socks or tights are prone to hygiene problems, especially in those who find that their feet perspire more than the average. The subject of excessively sweaty feet is covered fully on pages 45–6, but for everyone care in washing and drying the feet is important.

Wash the feet on a daily basis, and remember that this must be followed by careful drying, especially between the toes – an area which is often forgotten. If the skin is prone to be moist between the toes, wiping regularly with surgical spirit, plus a light powdering with talcum powder, will usually improve the situation.

Those people who have the reverse problem – a very dry skin – may find the application of a moisturising cream around areas of callous, nails and the heels beneficial. In the older person, whose skin will be naturally drier than a young person's, the frequency of washing the feet can be reduced to three or four times a week without causing hygiene problems, providing care is taken to keep the areas between the toes clean and dry.

The use of scrapers, etc. to reduce callous, apart from pumice stone or emery boards, is generally to be discouraged because of the dangers of damaging the skin. If a corn or callous requires more than gentle treatment with a pumice stone, then professional help from the chiropodist is probably required.

NAIL CARE

The toenails and their problems are dealt with in detail in Chapter 4. However, even normal healthy nails need care when cutting.

The nails should be cut straight across, although a slight contour can be made to follow the curve of the top of the toe.

They should not, however, be shaped as much as fingernails and certainly no attempt should ever be made to cut down the side of the toenail. This is the most common cause of a true ingrowing toenail, which is a very painful condition.

Some people never cut their nails but instead peel them to shorten them which is bad practice and can also lead to ingrowing nails. And no attempts should be made to clear out the sides of the toenails with any sharp or pointed implements.

The use of a stiff nailbrush to brush out any dead skin and nail debris when the skin is soft during a bath can be very beneficial for those who have problems with hard skin down the sides of their nails. However, the nail fold (cuticle) should never be interfered with, as pushing back this protective seal can allow infection to gain entry to the nail matrix area (the area from which nail grows).

A thickened toenail can be reduced in bulk by the use of a Diamond Deb nail rasp or an emery board, providing the problem is a minor one.

CLIMATE

Cold
The effects of cold on the feet can simply be uncomfortable, but for some individuals it can lead to the formation of chilblains or more serious problems (see page 76).

To minimise the effects of the cold make sure your footwear, including socks and tights, are insulating. The shoes or boots can have a thick sole, a fleecy lining or thermal-insulating insoles, while socks/tights can be made of materials, such as wool, which trap an insulating layer of air within their fibres. There must, however, be room within the shoes for this extra insulation, as a foot which is compressed in tight-fitting shoes will gain little benefit from thermal-insulating fleecy linings or insoles.

Hot
In hot weather it is important that your shoes should allow easy passage of air to the skin. Natural sweating will obviously take place over the surface of the foot, and this should be allowed to evaporate naturally into the atmosphere. The ideal footwear is the sandal but unfortunately this is not always a practical solution.

The use of contrast footbaths, one containing warm water and one containing cold water, in which you place the feet alternately, is often beneficial. It helps tone up the circulation, so relieving the congestion of blood and other tissue fluids in hot, tired, aching feet, although its effects are not likely to be very long-term.

PROBLEMS

Generally if you are concerned with any aspect of your foot health you should consult a chiropodist or your general practitioner for advice. However, if you should have an emergency problem, especially related to an infected/septic condition, then the following first aid measures may be helpful until professional help can be obtained.

Septic corns and other infected areas of the foot will generally benefit by placing the affected foot into a clean bowl containing warm water in which a handful of common household salt has been added. The foot should then be soaked for approximately 10–15 minutes. If the wound is open, discharge will flow out and will normally produce some relief from the pain. After the footbath the area should be carefully dried and then covered with a dry dressing (a sterile dressing such as Melolin can be purchased from the chemist) or a band-aid type of dressing.

The area should be rested, either totally – lying on the sofa with your feet raised – or by making sure no pressure falls on the area, which may mean cutting a hole in the shoe or slipper. As soon as possible treatment should be obtained from your chiropodist or doctor, especially if spread of infection is suspected – this will be indicated if the area of redness is increasing or if red lines radiate up into the leg.

EXERCISE IN BABIES

Before dealing with specific exercises, it is most important to mention the natural exercise that occurs in the first year of a child's life, which, if unwittingly or carelessly prevented, can have a marked effect on the healthy development of the feet. This kicking and flexing of the legs and feet is vital in order to develop the muscles, tendons and ligaments in these limbs. Attached to the developing bone structure, these components will, first of all, give the child the ability to stand, and this will soon be followed by the child's first steps. To ensure that these milestones are reached to the timetable determined by nature some simple rules need to be followed.

Allow the baby plenty of kicking time, preferably with the nappy (diaper) off, but certainly with the legs and feet uncovered. Stimulate the feet and legs by tickling or stroking them to encourage the baby to flex their new muscles.

Ensure that all-in-one suits are long enough in the legs to allow the baby's legs to stretch to their full length and that the feet of the garment are bigger than those of the baby without the material stretching. Similarly, check that socks are big enough to accommodate the feet without over-stretching. And never tuck the bedclothes in so tightly that the baby cannot move. Much of the baby's exercise is actually taken when they are 'resting' in their cot or pram.

Avoid baby walkers. It is much better for the baby to experience the natural stages that lead to walking rather than have an artificial means of getting around. A baby's natural curiosity in their surroundings gives them a major incentive to crawl or walk to whatever interests them. By introducing an artificial means you take away the need to learn these skills and the walking process may be slowed down.

FOOT EXERCISES

Most babies are born with healthy feet. If respected and treated well these feet will remain healthy throughout life. Exercise will help them stay this way.

There are almost no limits to what we can achieve with our feet. Indeed there are many people who, lacking the use of their arms and hands, are as capable of performing almost any task with their feet as a person without these handicaps. This fact alone should encourage people to exercise their feet, as fit feet are a good foundation for a healthy body.

However, most medical opinion would agree that the majority of people, particularly adults, would benefit from more regular exercise. Whether this exercise is simply a brisk walk every day, a specific sport such as squash or tennis, or even marathon running, a common factor is the need for healthy feet in order to perform the chosen exercise. For this reason, just as a boxer would not consider preparing for a bout without specifically exercising the parts of his body he will be relying on, i.e. his hands, so exercising the feet will enable an individual to perform their chosen activity more successfully and more enjoyably.

For children, exercises encourage healthy development of the feet, and are especially useful in this TV age when more and more youngsters spend their leisure time in front of the TV or computer screen. What's more, these foot exercises can be fun and can encourage children to become involved in other forms of exercise.

As with any exercise, it is important not to attempt an excessive number of any one activity. The secret of effective exercise is a reasonable number of cycles performed regularly. With children especially it is important to emphasise the 'fun' of the activity, so that the exercises do not become a task.

The following exercises are not just for children – they can be attempted by everyone, young and old alike. Indeed, the older you are probably the more reason there is for taking up these exercises. Performed correctly and regularly they will help the feet to become stronger and more supple and enable the owner to enjoy a more active and enjoyable life.

Foot and toe drill
These two exercises help to stretch and move the feet and toes in all directions.

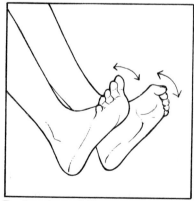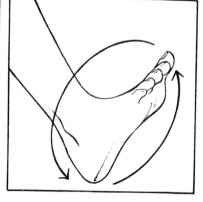

Foot and toe drill.

- Rest the feet on the heels, keeping them parallel to each other or with the toes turned slightly inwards. Flex, wriggle and extend the toes up to a maximum of 12 times.
- Starting with the foot at rest and at right-angles to the leg, extend the toes outwards, down and upwards as far as possible to complete a circle. Repeat this exercise up to 10 times for each foot, stretching it as far as possible each time.

Clock game

This exercise helps to strengthen and develop the muscles controlling the ankles.

Lying or sitting comfortably, stretch one leg out straight, point the toes and draw an imaginary circle by rotating the foot only, not the whole leg, in a clockwise direction. Complete six circles and then rotate the foot in the opposite direction. When completed repeat the exercise with the other foot.

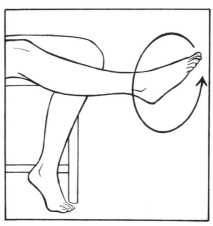

Clock game.

Walking the line

This is a simple exercise which, for children in particular, will help to improve their posture as they walk.

Draw a straight line on the floor and walk along it, pointing the toes down the line without falling off. Keep the back straight and the shoulders back, looking down the nose at the line to improve the posture.

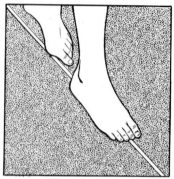

Walking the line.

Reefing the towel

This is an excellent exercise to develop strength and flexibility in the toes.

Stand on a towel with the heels touching one edge and the feet slightly turned in. Using the toes only, roll up the towel underneath the feet.

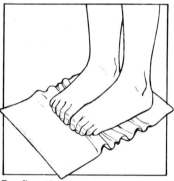

Reefing the towel.

Drawing with the toes

Not only does this exercise develop muscles and increase the suppleness of the toes but it increases the control of the foot in general.

Pick up a piece of chalk under the toes, not between them, and draw a picture with it. As the control of the foot improves the pictures will become more precise and more complicated drawings can be attempted.

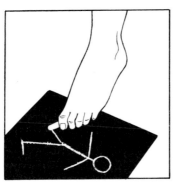

Drawing with the toes

The roller game

This exercise is particularly useful in developing the muscles of the inner longitudinal (lengthwise) arch which, although it need not be high to be healthy, may not get much exercise. This is particularly the case for women who wear high-heeled shoes; in such shoes the position of the foot is held constant and the movement of the arch is virtually nil.

Using a thin rolling pin or a piece of broom handle placed under the arches, roll it backwards and forwards for periods of a minute or longer. Repeat the exercise as often as you like, but don't overdo it as it may result in soreness under the arch.

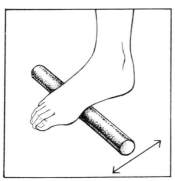

Roller game.

Counting toes

This is an exercise which stimulates the feet and encourages a good blood supply and suppleness.

Sitting on the floor or on a bed, extend the legs out straight

21

in front of you. Bend the right knee so that the foot is drawn up next to the left knee. Starting with the little toe, gently pull the toes to the right, one at a time, and massage the spaces between slowly and gently. Next, starting with the big toe, pull the toes gently to the left, one at a time, again massaging between the toes. Finally push each toe upwards and downwards as far as possible without causing any discomfort. Repeat with the left foot.

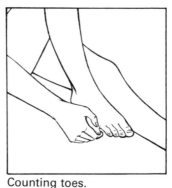

Counting toes.

Pony pawing

Another good exercise to develop strong ankles.

Standing on one foot, bend the knee of the other leg and point the toes of that foot towards the ground. Paw the ground with this leg just as a horse would. Repeat the exercise 12 times and then change over to the other leg.

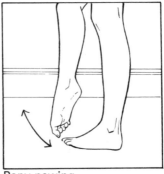

Pony pawing.

Marble race

A further exercise to develop the suppleness and flexibility of the toes, at the same time strengthening the ankles and legs and improving balance.

For this exercise you need some marbles and a dish. Standing in bare feet pick up a single marble with the toes, hop to the dish and drop the marble in. As the name suggests, this exercise can become a race by getting two or more people to participate. The race can be varied by increasing the number of marbles and/or increasing the distance between the pile of marbles and the dish.

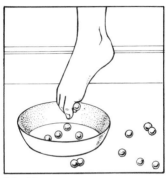

Marble race.

Pigeon parade

This exercise is for the sides of the foot and the ankles.

Standing, balance on the outer borders of the foot whilst raising the inner borders and slightly curling the toes in. Walk around in this position for up to one minute. Do not exceed this time or continue if painful as this may strain the foot.

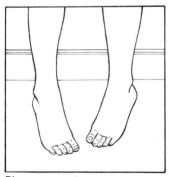

Pigeon parade.

Walking games

These are primarily for children and are designed to encourage a sense of balance and surefootedness.

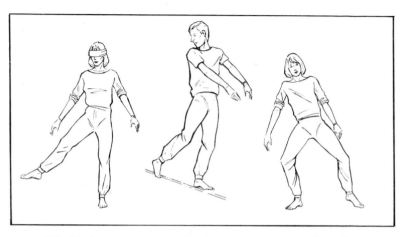

Blind balance.   Reverse.   Crab walk.

- **Blind balance** – in a large open space with no hazards or obstacles allow the child to walk wearing a blindfold and when this is mastered encourage them to balance on each foot in turn.
- **The reverse** – draw a straight chalk line and a large circle on the floor. First practise walking backwards along the straight line and then around the circle.
- **Crab walk** – stand up straight with the toes pointing forward. Keeping the toes in that direction walk sideways, first to the left then to the right.

FOOT HEALTH PROFESSIONALS

Sometimes, despite good general foot care, problems do arise which require medical attention. Health professionals who specialise in the treatment and care of the feet are known as chiropodists (in Britain) or podiatrists or podologists (in Australia, New Zealand, the United States, Canada, Europe, etc.).

The profession of chiropody or podology was, until the early 19th century, linked closely with dentistry, the same practitioner performing both skills. Gradually the two parted company, with little progression as far as chiropody was concerned until the beginning of the 20th century. The first school of chiropody opened in New York in 1912, followed in 1919 by the opening of the first school in Europe, the London Foot Hospital.

In most countries, chiropody is a closed profession, except in Britain where anyone can call themselves a chiropodist and practise without any training. However, to work for the national health service in Britain, practitioners must be state registered chiropodists (see pages 130–2 for more details). In this book, the word chiropodist will refer only to fully qualified and recognised practitioners, and for the sake of simplicity will cover the terms podologist and podiatrist.

In Britain, Australia and New Zealand the professions are very similar, apart from the name. However, in the USA, podiatrists have a longer training, with a greater emphasis on the surgical treatment of foot conditions, than their British, Commonwealth or European counterparts. Interestingly, some British chiropodists, especially those who have a particular interest in the surgical management of some foot problems, prefer to use the term podiatrist.

Orthopaedic surgeon

An orthopaedic surgeon specialises in the surgical treatment of bones and joints and is responsible for many of the operations on the foot. Surgery may not always be advisable and the orthopaedic surgeon may decide to refer you on to others in the health care team, such as the physiotherapist, chiropodist or the surgical shoemaker/orthotist.

3

FOOT PROBLEMS

INFLAMMATION

When the body's tissues are damaged in any way they will normally respond in a predictable manner. To begin with, more blood arrives at the site of injury, due to the local blood vessels dilating (opening out) more than usual. Fluid, and the body's protective white blood cells, then spread out from these dilated blood vessels into the damaged area.

As a result of this action four signs or symptoms are produced around the site of injury which, taken together, are known as inflammation:

- Redness
- Swelling
- Pain
- Heat

The redness and heat are produced by the increase in blood flow to the area, while the swelling is caused by fluid leaving the blood vessels and filling the tissues. The pain is the result of the extra fluid causing pressure on the nerve endings.

Inflammation is therefore a natural and essential part of healing, and will be seen in many of the following problems associated with the feet.

CALLOUS

A large proportion of foot problems in the adult are related to the skin's response to pressure and friction.

The skin's normal response to friction and pressure is to thicken, thus providing it with a means of protection. This is seen very clearly in the hands of a manual worker or an avid gardener; hard skin or callous forms on the palm near the base of the fingers. This same process can occur in the foot, especially on the sole of the foot in the region of the heads of the metatarsal bones, as well as on the tops and tips of the toes.

The cause is usually a problem with the shape or position of the foot and toes, combined with a shoe which is poorly styled or badly fitted. This hard skin initially is protective and is in many cases painless and trouble-free. However, in some people the build-up of callous goes beyond that required for pure protection and leads to pain and discomfort.

Removal of the callous by the chiropodist is quite painless and will provide immediate but short-term relief. If, however, the reason for the callous forming is not dealt with, its return is bound to occur. The problem may be aggravated by a slip-on court shoe in which the foot continuously slides forward during walking. A change in footwear may well lead to an improvement, with less callous being formed. A thin adhesive dressing covering the area may also help by reducing the friction and rubbing taking place on the skin.

If footwear is not the main problem then an insole or a device to improve the position and functioning of the foot and toes may be produced by the chiropodist.

CORNS

When the skin is compressed between two firm objects such as the shoe and bone, the skin will also respond by thickening. Usually in the centre of this thickening, where all the pressure meets, a hard central core will develop to produce a corn. A corn is therefore simply a concentrated area of hard skin, with no roots or living parts. Many people believe that a corn does have roots and that a cure cannot be achieved until these have been cut out and removed. When it is explained that it is just a hard core of impacted dead skin cells, most people seem quite disappointed!

The corn is usually found over a prominent and fixed joint of a toe, or on the sole of the foot in an area which is receiving an excessive amount of pressure. The nucleus of hard skin in the centre of the corn, which pinpoints the centre of pressure and stress, presses on nearby nerve endings to produce the characteristic stabbing pain of the corn.

An ordinary corn is the result of intermittent (on and off) pressure on the foot. However, if for some reason the pressure is constant and lasts for a long enough time, the tissues under the corn turn into a fluid and an ulcer will result. When removing the hard skin of a corn it is not uncommon to discover an ulcer with discharge underneath it. Many people presume that because there is discharge the corn is septic, but very often this is not the case; it is not actually infected and the problem is purely a mechanical one.

The main aim in treating a corn is to reduce the pressure over the affected area and redirect it to other parts which are better suited to take the loading. To achieve this, a protective pad using materials such as adhesive chiropody felt are applied around the corn. However, before the area is protected by such a pad, the excess skin and the central core of hard skin must be carefully removed by the chiropodist.

Self-treatment using a ring pad bought from a chemist may be useful, especially if the pad is cut so that it can be opened out to form a crescent. Medicated pads which produce a chemical burn are best not used, and in the elderly and diabetic they can produce serious consequences.

Removal of the cause is paramount if a permanent cure is to be achieved, and this will usually require either attention to the footwear, with regard to its style and fit, or an assessment of the foot's function during walking. If faulty foot function or bony deformities are the main problem, an insole or protective device can be produced by the chiropodist.

Corns are not all the same and can be divided into different types by the chiropodist.

Hard corn
The hard corn is the typical corn found on toes and underneath the metatarso-phalangeal joints and will always have a hard central core or nucleus, as described above.

Neurovascular corn
The neurovascular corn is a hard corn in which the blood vessels and nerves have become integrated into the hard skin.

It is therefore not only very painful but also liable to bleed easily, even during careful treatment by the chiropodist.

Treatment of this type of corn is not usually as successful as an ordinary hard corn and may require the use of electro-surgery or chemicals to remove the blood vessels and nerves which are complicating the condition.

Soft corn

Not all corns are hard; in fact some of them can be soft, these sort usually being located between the toes. In this position, because of sweat retention, they become waterlogged and rubbery. This soft rubbery corn can be just as painful as the worst hard corn, and because of its position it is often more difficult to treat.

Success in curing these corns is, however, high since the development of silicone rubber as a means of keeping the two bony parts of adjacent toes apart. The chiropodist can produce this toe wedge accurately moulded to the individual's toes and, providing skilful removal of the corn is performed, the corn should clear. When cure is not rapid the fault will normally lie with the patient's footwear or problems with the positions of toes in relation to each other.

Seed corns

In some people with dry skin, tiny corns, no more than 1 or 2 mm across, can occur on any part of the sole of the foot. They may in rare cases be linked with the same problem occurring in the palm of the hand in a condition known as keratoderma punctata.

Ordinary seed corns (they are a similar size to millet seeds) are seen just on the feet and may not necessarily be painful. If they are not too troublesome then a regular application of an emollient cream (such as Boots E45 or Aqueous Cream B.P.) will produce some benefit. When they are painful the removal of the overlying callous and each tiny plug of hard skin may be necessary, although a permanent cure to the problem is very unlikely.

Septic corn

A septic corn is an infected corn and means that a germ such as the bacteria *Staphylococcus aureus* has been able to penetrate the skin and damage the tissues. The body's response to an infection such as this is to protect itself by producing an inflammatory reaction. This means in the case of a septic corn that the area will become red, swollen, hot and painful.

There can be several reasons for the toe becoming septic. A common cause is the self-application of medicated corn plasters and ointments which contain an acid which loosens the skin and allows bacteria to enter. Similarly, constant pressure from shoes on one part of the foot will lead eventually to an ulcer forming. An ulcer is a break in the skin which is slow to heal, so very often these breaks will become infected by opportunist bacteria who are just waiting for this chance to invade the body. Self-treatment using blades and graters, or poor chiropody, can also be the cause of introducing sepsis.

Skilled treatment from the chiropodist is required to remove the overlying tissue, which will enable the discharge to be released and so relieve much of the pain. The area must then be cleaned, protected from pressure and an antiseptic dressing applied. The foot should be rested, and within a day or two most healthy individuals will find that the wound has healed and is no longer painful.

In some people, however, the infection does not respond in this way; instead the area becomes more swollen and the redness extends over a wider area. Sometimes red lines form, which run from the inflamed corn up the leg, and the glands at the back of the knee or in the groin may become swollen and painful. The red lines and pain in the glands all mean that the infection is spreading, and antibiotic treatment for the whole body will be needed quickly from your doctor if the condition is to be resolved.

THE BIG TOE

The big toe is known as the hallux and is composed of two bones known as phalanges. The joint between these two phalanges is therefore known as the inter-phalangeal joint. The phalanx in turn articulates with the first metatarsal and the joint between them, the metatarso-phalangeal joint, is very important but prone to problems.

BUNIONS

The most common problem is the bunion or hallux valgus, a condition in which the side of the big toe joint (the metatarso-phalangeal joint) becomes painful and enlarged.

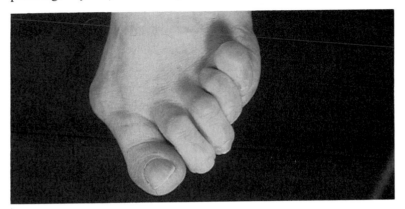

Bunion or hallux valgus.

To begin with, for various reasons detailed below, the big toe moves sideways towards the middle of the foot, which means that the joint is no longer articulating in a normal manner. Because of this position the side of the metatarsal is abnormally exposed, which produces a prominence on the side of the foot prone to pressure and friction from the shoe. The skin caught between the prominent joint and the shoe becomes damaged, and if this stress is a shearing one in which the foot is being rubbed by the shoe a bursa is formed. A bursa is a fluid-filled sac which is formed in the tissues under the skin; it is the body's method of protecting a bony prominence from friction, and it will fill up with fluid or reduce its fluid content depending on the stress which is stimulating it. When the bursa over the metatarsal head becomes full of fluid and inflamed the term bunion is often used, although the correct medical term would be bursitis.

As the big toe moves sideways, the other toes will be compressed and the result is usually that one of the toes moves out of the way. The second toe is the one usually squeezed out of position, and is forced to lie on top of the big toe. In this abnormal position the joint at the base of the toe – the metatarso-phalangeal joint – becomes partially dislocated.

This dislocation takes a long time to develop and cannot, unlike a dislocated shoulder or elbow, be pushed back into its normal position.

A second toe which is displaced by the big toe like this and becomes fixed is often referred to as a hammer toe. Because of its prominence, it is prone to trouble on its top (dorsal) surface, producing corns in response to the pressure and rubbing from the shoe. And this fixed position of the second toe also causes problems on the sole of the foot, often leading to corns and callous over the region of the second and third metatarsal heads.

As well as the problems with the big toe and the second toe, there is usually an associated widening of the foot across the metatarsal head region. This splaying of the forefoot leads to further problems with regard to shoe fitting as it becomes difficult to accommodate such a wide foot in a normal shoe.

The big toe's movement towards the middle of the foot is very often accompanied by the little toe (fifth toe) also moving towards the middle of the foot. This results in a 'bunion' on the outer (lateral) side of the foot over the fifth metatarso-phalangeal joint and is often referred to as a 'bunionette' or a tailor's bunion (the last name being given because it would often occur in tailors who in ages past sat cross-legged while working and so put excessive pressure on the outer borders of their feet).

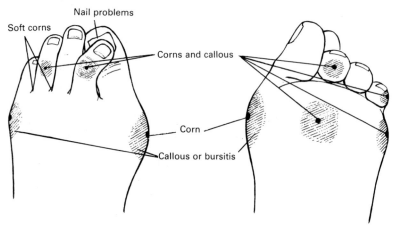

Hallux valgus with hammer second toe and other common problems on the top and sole of the foot.

32

It can be seen therefore that a sufferer with hallux valgus or bunions is likely to have more than a straightforward problem with one part of their foot. The two illustrations show many of the potential problems that are likely to occur in a typical case.

Causes of hallux valgus

Certain types of feet are more prone to develop hallux valgus than others. A foot which appears flat and excessively pronates will often produce an unstable foot which can lead to damage, resulting in the big toe being slowly pushed out of its normal position. The length of toes and the shape of the forefoot, factors inherited from our parents, can also make some people more susceptible than others.

Footwear is an additional important contributing factor as a pointed court shoe on a developing foot will obviously lead to the toes becoming wedge-shaped and the big toe being pushed over.

Treatment

The onset of the condition is usually painless and is likely to develop slowly, possibly starting in the young child or adolescent. Footwear advice at this stage is helpful to reduce the damaging influence of some shoes on the developing foot. Also an insole which reduces the excessive foot pronation may be used in the young adult to improve the foot's function and reduce the damage which otherwise might develop.

However, once hallux valgus is established in the adult foot it cannot be realigned and straightened, unless done surgically, as all the structures around the joint – the ligaments, tendons and bone surfaces – adapt to its abnormal position and no amount of exercise or manipulation will push it back. The chiropodist can help, however, in several ways to keep the foot comfortable and free from pressure over problem areas.

Finding a shoe to accommodate the wider foot is likely to be a problem, and it may be necessary for parts of the shoe to be specially stretched in the toe box to allow for a hammer toe, or it may be possible for a shoemaker or a chiropody appliance laboratory to modify the front of a shoe to provide more space.

The problems of corns over the prominent joints may be helped by the chiropodist making a protective device which fits onto the toe and around the painful joint. This is usually made first as a temporary pad stuck onto the skin, and then a more permanent but removeable device using silicone or latex rubber is produced for long-term protection.

Surgical treatment to straighten the big toe and the hammer second toe may be necessary for patients with severe deformities. However, as there have been over 100 different operations described for the treatment of hallux valgus over the years, only the most common will be described. A common procedure is known as a Keller's arthroplasty, in which a piece of the proximal phalanx bone is removed, plus a small section of the metatarsal head and the overlying bursa if present. This allows the toe to be straightened but produces a shortened and floppy toe. A recent innovation is to insert an artificial joint between the metatarsal and the shortened phalanx which helps retain the toe's length and enables it to function more normally.

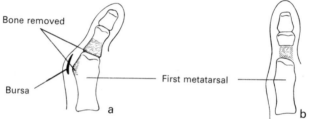

Keller's arthroplasty.

An osteotomy can also be performed on the shaft of the metatarsal, where a wedge of bone is removed which allows the bone to be straightened without interfering with the joint. A minor procedure for a less severe deformity could be to trim away the bony enlargement of the metatarsal head plus the bursa which narrows the foot slightly, although the problem can recur at a later stage.

A hammer second toe can also be straightened by surgery and it is usually sensible to have its position corrected at the same time as the big toe.

HALLUX RIGIDUS

A common condition affecting the big toe is the loss of movement in the joint (the first metatarso-phalangeal joint) which is known as hallux rigidus or hallux limitus. This joint is an important one for normal walking and running, and any major reduction in its ability to bend will cause problems elsewhere in the foot.

The reason for the toe becoming less mobile is usually because of osteo-arthritic changes which have taken place within the joint. The big toe should be able to bend upwards at the metatarso-phalangeal joint in a child by approximately 90 degrees. This wide range of movement is not necessary for the

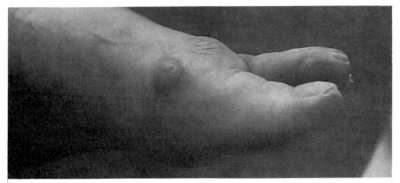

Hallux rigidus.

less active older person, but when movement is reduced to less than 20 degrees then problems are likely to arise.

The arthritic changes may be due to cartilage disorders which take place during growth or as a result of trauma. The trauma to the joint may be a single major episode or could be the result of repeated minor damage caused by continual stubbing of the big toe in a shoe which is fitted too short. The process of the joint becoming less mobile may be extremely painful and may be extended over a period of months or years. In some cases, however, a very stiff joint can arise having caused little or no pain in its development. Once the joint has become fixed it is usually no longer painful.

During the painful stages the female patient will soon learn that the heel height of her shoe has an effect on the comfort of the joint. As the heel height increases, so the big toe is jarred upwards; when the toe is jarred upwards to its maximum it is likely to be at its most painful. The heel height must therefore be reduced, until very often only a flat or low-heeled shoe can be tolerated. And even the stiff painless joint is not without its problems. Because the big toe joint is a major bending point of the foot during walking, an alternative bending point must be found, and the small joint in front of it within the toe, known as the inter-phalangeal joint, has to compensate; it develops more mobility than nature intended and will often adopt a hyper-extended position which leads to the toenail becoming compressed by the toecap of the shoe.

The skin under the inter-phalangeal joint of the big toe will often respond to this additional workload by thickening and producing callous and corns. Likewise the outer border of the foot takes more of the load during walking and may develop skin thickening or corns. The big toe joint itself will become larger because of the arthritic changes which have taken place within it. The top (dorsal) part of the joint will often have a bony ridge which can be seen and felt; if this bony outgrowth is large enough it may rub on the shoe and lead to problems with an inflamed bursa or painful corns.

Treatment

In the acute or early stages ice packs massaged around the joint to relieve the pain should be beneficial. It may be helpful if the chiropodist uses strapping to reduce the amount of movement in the joint on a short-term basis, until the joint settles down. Then, as the pain reduces, ultrasound and manipulation by the chiropodist or physiotherapist is usually helpful. Also, at this stage, footwear advice and an assessment of the sufferer's foot function may be useful in order to reduce any aggravating factors.

During the chronic or later stages, as the joint becomes fixed, the pain normally reduces, although the resulting foot problems may well need treating. A shoe insert to reduce the amount of pressure on any painful areas, plus removal of the thickened skin by the chiropodist, may be all that is necessary. It may be possible, although not always acceptable to the sufferer, to adapt the shoe by making the sole rigid and curved (a wooden clog is a classic example), thus enabling the person to walk without bending and stressing the foot.

It may be necessary to intervene surgically with the big toe joint, either by providing a new joint with a silicone-rubber implant (an arthroplasty) or by fixing the joint (arthrodesis) in a suitable position for footwear. The surgical fixing of the joint will not necessarily have beneficial effects on the loading on other joints and could in fact lead to problems with, for instance, the inter-phalangeal joint of the big toe.

THE HIGHLY-ARCHED FOOT

Although the flat foot can produce many problems, a high-arched foot (pes cavus, from the Latin *pes* = foot, *cavus* = cavity) can be just as much of a problem, but for different reasons. This type of foot can be inherited or may be a consequence of muscle and nerve imbalance, being seen in such neurological conditions as poliomyelitis and spina bifida. In a severe case an arch will be seen along the length of both the inner (medial) and outer (lateral) borders of the foot. (An arch across the forefoot (metatarsal arch) is not seen in a normal weight-bearing foot so the mythical dropped metatarsal arch is not considered to exist nowadays.)

In the high-arched foot the toes too are usually affected as they are clawed and do not touch the ground when standing, which produces a foot whose only contact with the ground is the heel and the metatarsal heads. The foot will often be stiff and unable to function efficiently, resulting in corns and callous forming on the skin over the metatarsal heads. The patient will also often complain of discomfort in the tight ligaments and tissues which connect the forefoot with the heel as well as problems where their clawed toes are rubbed by the shoe.

Treatment

In the young patient, with movement still available in the toes and metatarso-phalangeal joints, it may be helpful to keep these joints mobile with stretching exercises. Careful choice of footwear is important, and socks or tights that do not restrict and therefore do not aggravate clawing of the toes should be worn.

In the foot which is no longer mobile it is possible to provide comfort for the patient by producing a custom-made insole which helps to take the pressure from the small overloaded areas to other areas more suited to taking the load. Footwear which is deep enough to accommodate the toes will not be easy to find, but it is necessary, otherwise the shoe will press on the tops of the toes, causing pressure problems.

In severe cases surgery can be performed to the soft tissues such as tendons and ligaments to lengthen them. Wedges of bone can also be removed from the middle of the foot which may then allow the foot to flatten.

FLAT FOOT

Ideally the height of the long arch of the foot should vary during walking. When you are standing with your weight directly over your feet the long arch will be at its lowest. The foot is said to be pronated when it is in this position; it is in its most flexible state. The arch will be at its highest when you raise your heel and go onto tiptoe. The foot is then said to be supinated; it is an important position in walking as it provides the rigid lever you need to propel yourself along.

Some feet, even on tiptoe, do not form a long arch and these can be called true flat feet or pes planus. This type of foot is often inherited and, surprisingly, causes few serious problems to the owner, apart from a somewhat inelegant style of walking. It is not possible to correct this type of foot shape by surgery, and insoles to support a non-existent arch generally have no therapeutic value.

The foot type which causes more trouble than the true flat foot is the one which excessively pronates, or pronates when it should be supinating. This means that the arch will be low and the foot flexible when it should be rigid and highly arched. The consequence of having a mobile foot when it should be rigid is that the foot will be easily damaged by the footwear, which can then lead to conditions such as bunions, claw toes, corns and callous. It will also put strain on the soft tissues under the foot so that pain in the long arch and the heel area can arise.

The reasons for the foot to be pronating when it should not are varied and complex. Problems at the hip, knee and ankle can all have an effect on the foot, causing it to pronate abnormally. However, it is also common for a foot problem to produce a pronating foot which in turn causes pain and other problems in the knee, hip and back. By careful examination the chiropodist can assess from where the problem originates. Is it just a leg problem, a foot problem or is it a combination of both?

In suitable cases it is possible to produce an insert for the shoe (an orthosis) which enables the foot to function more normally and reduces the amount of damaging pronation. This orthosis has to be made very accurately on a cast of the patient's foot. It is usually made from a plastic material which is heat moulded to the patient's cast and then 'balanced' by adding or grinding away areas of the device, which then fills in the space between the foot and the ground when walking. An orthosis made in this way has a very different function and effectiveness than the plastic and metal arch-supports which are mass produced and sold in chemists and similar shops. Flat feet in children is dealt with separately – see pages 60–1.

PLANTAR DIGITAL NEURITIS

This condition, often known as Morton's toe, produces pain, starting in the area of the cleft of the third and fourth toe, which radiates up into the fourth toe. It may start as a tingling burning sensation that develops into a severe stabbing pain which shoots up to the end of the toe. Sometimes the pain is less severe and produces a pins-and-needles sensation which makes the toe feel numb. The pain occurs in walking, usually in women, and the sufferer will often try to relieve the discomfort by removing the shoe and massaging the area near the fourth toe. Other toes may be affected, but this is much less common.

The reason for the pain is still a matter of debate. The nerve close to the area of pain will often appear thickened and surrounded by fibrous tissue, which is known as a neurofibroma. Many different theories exist, popular ones being irritation of the thickened nerve by pressure from the metatarsal heads, reduction in the blood supply to the nerve, and irritation of the bursa between the metatarsal heads.

Footwear advice is often required as the condition is usually seen in conjunction with the wearing of constricting court shoes with an inadequate depth and width. The other important factor is that usually the fastening of the shoe is inadequate or totally lacking, so ideally the sufferer should change to a well-fitted shoe with a lace or buckle that holds the foot within the shoe.

Padding in the form of toe props to improve the position of the toes, plus protective padding for the underneath of the foot, may be required. These can be provided as short-term adhesive pads initially and then transferred into more durable devices if long-term management is needed.

If footwear advice and corrective devices do not relieve the symptoms then surgery may be required to remove the thickened nerve.

ATHLETE'S FOOT

This common infection of the skin (also called *Tinea pedis*) is caused by a fungus which lives on the protein, keratin, which is found in the outer layers of the skin. These fungi that live on the skin are called dermatophytes (derm = skin, phytes = plants) and belong to several different families, so their effect on the skin and the subsequent symptoms will vary. The infection is thought to be transferred from the infected skin cells of one individual to another from the floor surfaces upon which bare feet come into contact, e.g. swimming baths, changing rooms, etc.

The most common site of infection is between the toes, where the dark, warm and moist conditions encourage the fungus to colonise and eventually to spread out to surrounding areas. The most obvious sign of infection is an edge of scaly, loose skin forming a ring around an area of pink denuded skin. In between the toes this scaling is often accompanied by an area of white soggy water-laden skin. This macerated skin may simply be an effect of excessive sweating (see hyperhidrosis on page 45), but is more often associated with a fungus infection.

At the base of the toe there may also be a moist split in the skin (a fissure). This fissure may be deep enough to cause slight bleeding, or may become secondarily infected with a bacteria which can cause inflammation (redness, swelling and pain) plus discharge. A fungus infection on its own does not cause inflammation or discharge, the only symptoms usually being an itching irritation.

To confirm a diagnosis of fungus infection it may be necessary for the chiropodist or dermatologist to send a sample of the loose scaly skin to a laboratory for investigation. Under the microscope the tiny threads of fungus can be seen and by allowing it to grow on a culture plate the organism can be identified exactly.

Fungi can also infect other parts of the foot apart from between the toes. It can cause scaling and the formation of tiny blisters accompanied by itching, especially along the inner long arch of the foot and around the heel. One particular type of fungus, *Trichophytum rubrum*, can cause a rather different reaction by making the sole of the foot and toes seem extremely dry, with white chalky lines along the skin creases.

This infection is probably the most difficult one to treat successfully. It is possible for fungi that normally affect household pets such as cats and dogs also to affect humans. Although not common, such an infection will tend to cause more severe symptoms of inflammation and irritation than the normal ones that affect humans.

Another type of organism, classified as a fungus but not a dermatophyte, is the yeast called *Candida albicans* which can affect skin and nails. It is the same organism that causes thrush and is seen sometimes as an infection in the skin folds around the fingernails and, occasionally, the toenails. Unlike the fungi that produce athlete's foot, it can produce inflammation, pain and a yellow discharge.

Treatment

The treatment of athlete's foot is often protracted and unsuccessful, despite the fact that in recent years some very effective fungicides have been produced. A group of drugs known as the imidazoles can now be purchased by the public or can be obtained on prescription. Trade names of some of the common ones are Daktarin, Canestan and Ecostatin and they can be purchased as creams, lotions and powders. There are less expensive alternatives such as Tinaderm, Tineafax, Mycil, Mycota, etc., which may be more readily available and which in some cases work effectively.

The main problem in treatment is that people do not treat the infected area for long enough. The cream or ointment will be diligently applied while the skin is itchy and peeling, but as soon as the skin looks normal and symptoms disappear the applications will dwindle to a dose 'now and then'. The problem is that the fungus can reproduce as a spore, similar to a seed, which can lie dormant on the skin for long periods. When a fungicidal cream is applied it produces unfavourable conditions for the fungus, which will appear to have been eradicated. However, spores may well have been produced and when the cream is discontinued conditions will probably revert back to those favourable to the fungus and the spores will release new fungi to spread and invade the skin again.

It is, however, very difficult to persuade a patient that application of the fungicide for several weeks or months, after all symptoms have disappeared, is necessary for a condition which is seldom more than a minor irritation. Once the problem seems resolved an application of fungicidal dusting powder lightly applied to the spaces between the toes and in the patient's socks or tights is likely to be beneficial in the long-term management of the condition. A very simple remedy of applying surgical spirit between the toes may often change the quality of the skin so that the fungus no longer finds it a favourable home. The spirit needs to be applied on a regular basis to provide any benefit and may initially cause some discomfort if applied to splits (fissures) which are commonly found in the skin between the toes.

The same fungi that affect the skin can also invade and colonise the toenails and this is discussed fully in Chapter 4.

THE HEEL

The heel comes under a great deal of stress during walking and running and has a thick layer of fatty tissue under the heel bone to act as a shock absorber.

Heel callous
The skin around the edge of the heel will often become thickened and sometimes painful. The reason may be very simple; for example, the wearing of sling-back shoes or sandals will tend to irritate the edge of the heel and so promote the production of callous. Also the heel seat of many court shoes will be too small for the person's heel, with the result that the skin is pinched and irritated at the groove where the upper of the shoe meets the inner sole.

A change in the style of footwear and the use of an emery board or pumice stone will usually rectify the problem.

Heel fissures
In a person with dry skin (anhidrosis) the edge of the heel may be the site of splits in the skin known as fissures. If these are not too deep, a vigorous regime of applying a moisturising cream such as E45 or Aqueous Cream B.P. regularly on a daily basis will be helpful. This treatment will usually clear up superficial fissuring, but sometimes the fissures are deeper, causing pain and bleeding.

Careful treatment is required to remove the callous from the edge of the fissure which will assist it to heal. The chiropodist may also apply an antiseptic emollient in the form of an ointment or an impregnated gauze. Adhesive strapping around the heel may be required to stop the skin from being pulled apart and so allow normal healing to take place. Long-term treatment may need the making of a rubber heel-cup, made on a cast of the patient's heel, which retains the body's moisture and keeps the skin moist and supple.

Dry skin elsewhere on the foot will also benefit from regular applications of a moisturising cream and in bad cases a cream known as Calmurid (10 per cent urea cream) is very effective.

Heel pain

Pain in the heel can be due to an inflamed bursa, either under the heel or at the back of the heel where the Achilles tendon joins the heel bone. The inflamed bursa under the heel, sometimes known as postman's or policeman's heel, is usually the result of excessive walking or running and if rested will normally resolve itself, although if necessary a cushioning heel pad can be provided.

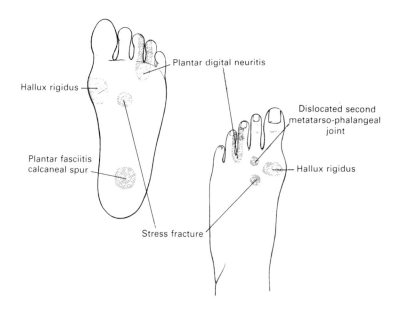

Common sites of pain on the sole and top of the foot.

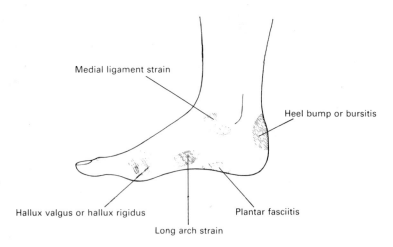

Medial ligament strain

Heel bump or bursitis

Hallux valgus or hallux rigidus

Plantar fasciitis

Long arch strain

Common sites of pain in the medial (inner) side of the foot.

At the back of the heel (retro-calcaneal) there are two bursae which can cause problems if irritated by the heel counter of the shoe. The back of the heel will then become red and swollen and when you press it you will be able to feel the fluid inside moving.

Treatment in the early stages to reduce the inflammation will involve the use of cooling lotions such as witch hazel or ice packs. The heel counter of the shoe, which is often too hard or badly shaped, can be softened with a hammer so that it becomes pliable and less likely to dig into the heel bone. Raising the heel using a sponge or felt pad may alter the positions of the conflicting parts of the foot and shoe and therefore improve matters.

PLANTAR FASCIITIS

This is a pain in the tough fibrous band that connects the heel bone to the fore-part of the foot. Damage can occur to the area where this fibrous band joins the bone, and this in turn can produce an inflammatory condition of the heel. During the process of inflammation a ridge of extra bone may be laid down on the under-surface of the heel bone and this can be seen in an X-ray, resembling a spur or spike. However this spur on the calcaneum is usually the result of the heel pain rather than its cause; when the other foot is also X-rayed, a calcaneal spur which is quite symptom-free will often be seen. The cause of plantar fasciitis/calcaneal spur is unclear but very often the patient is over 50 and cannot remember any damage to their foot which could explain the problem. In a few cases there will be a history of arthritic problems such as Reiter's syndrome and ankylosing spondylitis.

The description of the pain is usually very similar in all cases, the patient finding the heel most painful after a period of rest, perhaps after sitting watching the television or first thing in the morning when weight is put on the affected foot. After walking for a short period the pain usually decreases and becomes bearable, although by the end of a busy day it is likely to be constantly painful. The site of the pain can vary from the very centre of the sole (plantar) surface of the heel to a point around the edge of the heel or along the fibrous band of the plantar fascia itself in the area of the long arch of the foot.

Treatment
The chiropodist is usually able to help by providing an insole which reduces the strain on the plantar fascia and re-directs pressure away from the painful spot, whilst providing some cushioning and comfort to the heel. This padding may be assisted by the application of ultrasound, which helps reduce the pain and resolve the inflammation. Steroid injections are sometimes used and provide temporary relief for some people, although their long-term use is often disappointing.

SWEATY FEET

Sweaty feet (hyperhidrosis) may be a source of humour to some people, but for the sufferer it can be a most distressing problem.

The production of sweat is a natural process, important in keeping the skin at an even temperature. The skin on the sole of the foot and the palms of the hand has a greater number of sweat glands than most other parts of the body. The sweat glands on the feet and hands also have another function, which is to react rapidly to emotional stress. This is seen most clearly in the clammy hands of the person being interviewed for a job or sitting an examination.

The problem of sweaty feet may be a true over-production of sweat, which will also be noticeable in the sufferer's hands, or it might be that the shoes or hosiery are made of materials that stop the natural process of evaporation of the sweat from the skin.

Whatever the reason for the problem, it will be important to ensure that the footwear is not aggravating the situation. The ideal material for the shoe upper is leather, which is capable of absorbing moisture which can then pass through the material and evaporate away. It is also important that the shoe lining is not a synthetic material such as nylon, which will prevent a leather upper absorbing the sweat, or that the leather is not made impermeable by applying a 'patent' leather finish to its outside. During the warmer weather a sandal can be worn by many people, which will allow the sweat to evaporate readily. If a closed-in shoe must be worn, then often two or three small holes punched in the upper near the instep area produce enough ventilation to prevent sweat retention.

The socks or tights worn by the sufferer can also effectively stop sweat from evaporating, especially when they are made of synthetic materials such as nylon. Therefore the best materials for hosiery are the natural ones such as wool and cotton, or even mixtures of natural and synthetic materials. The sufferer must also take care to change socks or tights daily, and if possible change the shoes as well, so that one pair can be drying out while another is being worn.

The skin can be wiped over daily with a preparation of surgical spirit after the feet have been washed and dried and then powdered lightly with a dusting powder. In severe cases it may even be necessary to change shoes and hose and wash the feet twice daily, although this can produce practical problems because of the sufferer's occupation or lifestyle.

Smelly feet

Sweat is an odourless fluid, but when left for a time on the skin it is affected by certain bacteria which then produce a rather unpleasant smell. The problem of smelly feet (bromidrosis) is usually connected with sweaty feet, and the odour produced will usually respond to the measures already outlined in the treatment above for sweaty feet.

Commercial insoles containing carbon, which are made to absorb gases and odour, can be useful, especially when combined with good hygiene and regular changing of footwear, etc. In some cases potassium permanganate crystals dissolved in water to produce a pink-coloured foot-bath can be beneficial if used on a regular basis.

MOLES

Most people have at least a dozen moles over their whole body and the vast majority of these are quite harmless. Some moles, however, can become malignant and turn into a harmful skin cancer which can send secondary cancers to other organs of the body. The moles on the foot and leg are sometimes affected in this way, so careful watch should be made of their size, colour and condition.

If a mole suddenly starts to increase in size, becomes itchy, bleeds or seems to be producing offspring, then the doctor should be notified quickly and if he thinks necessary you will be referred to the hospital dermatologist. When seen early enough these malignant melanomas can be cut out and their removal provides a permanent cure. If ignored then the growth will extend and have very serious consequences.

VERUCCAE

A verucca is a wart found on the sole of the foot. It is caused by the same virus which produces warts elsewhere on the body. As most people suffer from veruccae during childhood, more information on this problem can be found in Chapter 5 (pages 66–9).

4

THE TOENAIL

The toe and fingernails are highly specialised adaptions of the skin and are therefore prone to many of the problems which commonly affect the skin. The toenails have additional problems caused by the damage from shoes and from pressure.

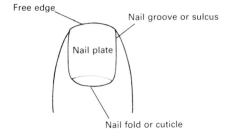

Toenail.

The area from which the nail grows is known as the nail matrix; it cannot be seen as it is under the nail fold. As it grows forward the nail is firmly attached to the tissue underneath, which is known as the nail bed. The end of the nail is known as its free edge, whilst its sides lie in the nail grooves or sulci.

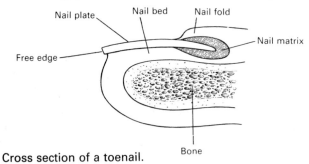

Cross section of a toenail.

The toenail is a very slow-growing structure, taking nine months to a year to grow from its base to its free edge. This process is quicker in young people, who also tend to have thinner nails than an elderly person.

CUTTING TOENAILS

Generally the idea is to cut the toenail straight across and never to cut down the sides. This is very sound advice, although there is no reason why the free edge of the nail should not follow the shape of the end of the toe. A nail that is cut straight across invariably leaves two sharp corners which, in the shoe, may dig into and cut adjacent toes.

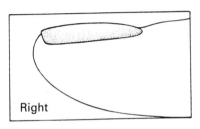 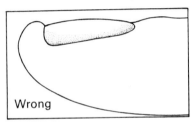

Correct length of a toenail.

Nails can be cut too short. This produces a problem for the nail plate as it grows forward as it has to push through the soft tissue which is pressed up against it.

And cutting a V shape into the middle of the nail to relieve pressure along the sides of the nail is a totally useless exercise, even though it is still recommended inadvisably for the treatment of an ingrowing toenail.

INGROWING TOENAIL

This is a term greatly misused by people who mistakenly think that the nail is ingrowing when really their problem is one of corns or callous developing down the sides of the nail.

A true ingrowing toenail (onychocryptosis) is when the side of the nail penetrates the skin of the nail groove. If left untreated this allows the entry of bacteria, and the area

49

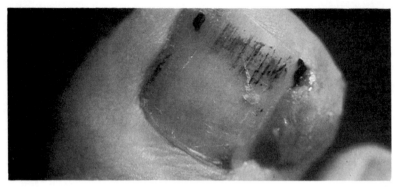

Ingrowing toenail.

becomes infected and inflamed. Also, if the nail remains embedded in the soft tissue the skin cannot heal over, and in its efforts to seal the wound it produces granulation tissue which becomes heaped up on the side and top of the nail plate. This excessive granulation tissue bleeds very easily and tends to obscure the site of the problem.

Young people in their teens and twenties are the group most affected. Some people will have a tendency to this problem if their nails are thin, brittle and break easily and if their skin is inclined to be moist. Cutting down the sides of the nail or cutting the nail too short can also start the problem. The condition is often extremely painful but happily its treatment should be both simple and effective.

In some the skilful removal of the small section of nail causing the problem can be undertaken without a great deal of discomfort, allowing the wound to heal. If the area is too sensitive, so that even the cleaning or swabbing of the toe is painful, a local anaesthetic given by the chiropodist will be required to enable the offending section to be removed.

In many cases, when the condition is severe or recurring, then the treatment of choice is likely to be partial nail avulsion with phenolisation of the nail matrix (the growing area of the nail). This complex-sounding procedure is always undertaken under local anaesthesia, so might be unsuitable where an injection is contra-indicated because of the patient's medical history. This is usually uncommon, but underlines the importance of always keeping the chiropodist up to date with your medical history, however unrelated to your foot problem it may seem.

In a partial nail avulsion the offending side of nail is removed and a chemical is applied to the cells which are responsible for producing the nail. After the procedure has been carried out it may take four to six weeks for the small wound to heal and during this time a dressing on the toe may be required until the wound becomes dry. The bulk of the nail plate is left intact and will appear cosmetically near normal. Providing all the nail cells have been destroyed, the offending section does not regrow and so the problems related to it cannot recur.

INVOLUTED TOENAIL

The normal nail plate has a slight curve from side to side and from front to back. In some people this curvature from side to side is so exaggerated that it produces pain down the sides of the nail and is known as an involuted toenail. Often this excessive curvature is also associated with the formation of corns or callous down the sides of the nail, which may lead to additional discomfort.

This type of nail can often be difficult to cut properly and there may be a temptation for people to cut down the sides of

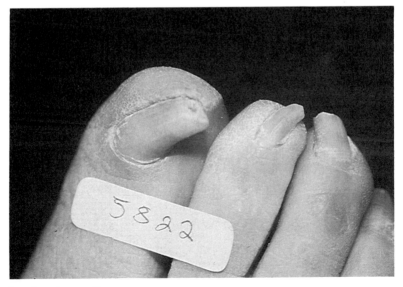

Involuted toenail.

their nails to relieve the discomfort that is occurring. This may give temporary relief, but as the nail grows forward it must now push its way through the soft skin at the side of the nail which has taken up the space previously occupied by the nail. This sequence of events will in some cases lead to a true ingrowing toenail and require minor surgical treatment, as mentioned previously.

In many cases of involuted toenail, though, it is possible for the chiropodist to clear the side of the nail of corn and callous and reshape the side of the nail slightly. The side can then be packed with a material such as foam or small plastic gutters which act as a barrier between the hardness of the nail and the soft tissue around it. It is also possible to improve the shape of the nail and reduce its tendency to curve at the sides by applying a small stainless steel wire brace to the nail.

All these methods of treatment, however, will have little long-term benefit if footwear is allowed to pinch the toes and so compress the soft tissues and the sides of the nails together. And if all these measures fail to relieve the patient's problem it may be advisable to remove the side of the nail or the whole nail plate and stop the nail from regrowing.

THICKENED TOENAIL

A very common condition affecting the toenails of many elderly people is the thickened nail (onychogryphosis). There are several causes of nail thickening but the most common is that of damage to the area of the nail which produces the nail

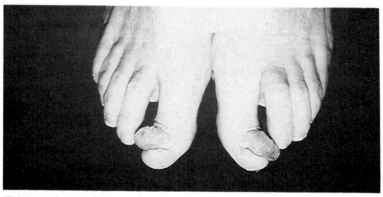

Thickened toenail.

cells. The damage can be caused by a major trauma such as a heavy weight falling onto the nail, or by minor stress which occurs over many years when the toenail is persistently stubbed against the end of the shoe. Once damaged, the thickening of the nail is irreversible and as it grows forward it will usually curve and produce what is known as a ram's-horn nail.

Although very distressing to the patient, this type of nail problem is very easy to treat. The thickness of the nail can be reduced quite painlessly by the use of a small electric drill. The improved appearance and the relief from pain is immediate and often spectacular. However, as the condition is irreversible the nail will in time revert back to its distorted form, so routine reduction of its thickness is likely to be required every two or three months.

In a young patient, when only one or two nails are thickened, a total nail avulsion in which the damaged nail is removed and treated so that it does not regrow may be advisable.

If a thickened toenail is left untreated, the bulk of the nail in the confines of the shoe's toebox can cause so much pressure on the nail bed that it softens and liquefies. This can lead to an ulcer forming under the nail which, in a patient with poor circulation, could produce serious complications.

FUNGAL INFECTION OF THE TOENAIL

It is also possible for a nail to become thickened due to an infection by a fungus which invades the nail plate and lives within it or under it. As well as becoming thickened, the texture of the nail also changes as it becomes crumbly, whilst its colour may vary from white to a dark brown. This condition, known as onychomycosis, is usually seen in conjunction with a fungal infection of the skin (athlete's foot), and can affect just one nail or all of them.

Unfortunately the treatment of an infection of the toenail such as this is both long and often unsuccessful. The length of time it takes to treat the nail is protracted because the toenail grows so slowly (nine months-plus for a completely new nail to regrow) and the infection needs to grow out with the nail before one can be satisfied that it is clear of fungus.

Another factor affecting treatment is that fungicidal creams or lotions which are painted onto the nail have to penetrate very deeply to the cells underneath the nail plate if they are to work effectively. This is only likely to occur if the thickness of the nail can be reduced to almost the nail bed. The ideal method is to have the nail thickness reduced professionally by the chiropodist every two to three months. Alternatively the sufferer can use a file or rasp themselves to keep the nail reduced; however, this must be done sensibly as the rasp, once used on an infected nail, can then be responsible for transferring the infection to a normal nail if it is not sterilised in between.

Creams and lotions which can be recommended by the chiropodist or doctor might include preparations such as Daktarin, Canestan, Phytex, etc. There are alternative treatments for onychomycosis, using tablets such as griseofulvin or ketoconazole, but their success on toenails, unlike fingernails and skin, is often disappointing and the occasional side effects make doctors cautious with regard to their use for toenail infections.

If only one toenail is affected the chiropodist may advise removal of the nail under local anaesthesia and the application of a suitable fungicide as the new nail grows forward. This is usually more successful than applying the external agent to the intact infected nail, but is a rather radical treatment for a condition which seldom causes the patient any serious problems.

OTHER CAUSES OF NAIL THICKENING

Apart from damage-induced (onychogryphosis) and fungal-infected (onychomycosis) nails, several other reasons for the nails to thicken can be found. Psoriasis is a condition which produces skin problems in the form of a scaly rash and, in some individuals, joint problems. It can produce a thickened nail with, in some instances, small 'thimble' pits on its surface. The nails generally do not produce painful problems for the sufferer but may need reducing in bulk by the chiropodist in order to improve their comfort.

Other conditions which produce or are thought to produce an increase in the thickness of the nail include dermatosis and circulatory problems.

SUB-UNGUAL HAEMATOMA

A blood blister under the toenail is a common occurrence and is usually the result of injury, possibly by someone stepping on the affected nail or by dropping a heavy weight on it. The same effect will result from stubbing the toe against a hard object or from the impact on the toe caused by certain sports such as sprinting, soccer, squash, etc.

The damage to the nail causes the tiny blood vessels under the nail plate to break so that bleeding occurs between the nail bed and the nail plate. The blood cannot normally escape so it causes a build-up of pressure on the nerve endings, which in turn produces a great deal of pain. In some cases the damage causes the whole nail plate to separate and shed, thus allowing the blood to escape and, as a consequence, reducing the pain.

If the nail is seen shortly after the damage has occurred and the blood is still trapped under the plate, it may be advisable to reduce the pressure by making two small drainage holes in the nail plate. This can be achieved by using a needle or wire (a straightened-out paper-clip will even do) which is heated until red hot in a flame. If this is gently placed on the nail plate it will burn a small hole through it. Two holes are required, on the same principle which applies to opening a tin of evaporated milk or a beer can. The fluid when free will readily soak into cotton wool, and when drained the area should be kept covered and clean for a few days until the area is completely dry.

For those who are unable or unwilling to attempt such self-treatment the chiropodist can relieve the pressure by making two small holes in the nail plate using an electric drill, but this must be done before the blood under the nail has had time to clot and harden.

Because the seepage of blood will have separated the close relationship between the cells of the nail bed and the nail plate, incomplete shedding of the nail may result. This means that a large part of the nail is detached from the nail bed and may need trimming to reduce the problems of it catching on socks or tights whilst other parts are firmly attached. The nail must completely regrow before a normal-looking appearance returns.

SUB-UNGUAL EXOSTOSIS

A small bony lump (exostosis) may occasionally grow from the bone at the end of the toe (the distal phalanx as it is called), under the toenail. As the bony lump enlarges, the soft tissue between the bone and the nail becomes compressed. The nail will usually become distorted by the exostosis and the effect of a shoe pressing on the nail produces a painful problem. The cause may be difficult to identify, although a history of injury or continuous pressure from footwear may be given.

Temporary relief can be given by the chiropodist with protective padding, reduction of the nail's thickness, and footwear advice, but long-term treatment will usually require the surgical removal of the exostosis.

PARONYCHIA

This means inflammation of the nail and the surrounding area, and the condition may have several different causes.

- Infection, which may be linked with poor nail-cutting or a true ingrowing toenail.
- Repeated damage from the shoe irritating and compressing the soft tissues around the nail.
- A *Candida albicans* infection, which is more likely to affect fingernails than toenails.

Treatment of paronychia will depend on the cause and will therefore vary in each case.

OTHER MEDICAL PROBLEMS

The nail, like the skin, is affected by many general health problems and in some instances is used as a diagnostic aid during the clinical examination of a patient. By looking at the shape of a fingernail or toenail the medical specialist may be given a clue to the health of the patient. The following conditions are examples of the link between the nail and other medical problems.

Koilonychia

In this condition the nail loses its normal contour so that it becomes flat or concave (spoon-shaped). This is seen more often in the fingernails than the toenails and is often associated with iron-deficiency anaemia.

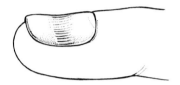

Koilonychia.

Onycholysis

This means the separation of the nail from the nail bed, starting at the free edge. A common cause is pressure from shoes, etc., but it is also seen in such conditions as psoriasis, dermatitis, poor circulation and thyroid disorders.

Beau's lines

This is a ridge or depression across the nail plate of all the nails, caused by an interference in the nutrition to the nail. It is often associated with such conditions as measles, mumps, pneumonia and heart disease. A ridge across a single nail is more likely to be caused by pressure damage. Whatever the cause, the nail will usually grow out normally.

Clubbing of nails

This is an exaggerated curvature of the nail from the matrix to the free edge. The condition affects the ends of the fingers and toes making them enlarged, which has an effect on the shape of the nail. The term 'drumstick' is sometimes used to describe the condition, because of its appearance. Clubbing is often associated with chronic respiratory and heart disease.

Onychorrhexis

In this condition, otherwise known as brittle nail, the nail plate is thinner than normal and may have ridges or splits running along the length of the nail. These nails are brittle and will easily crack, producing a rough free edge, but otherwise are not likely to produce any serious problems.

The cause may be one of a lowered general health, certain skin diseases, anaemia, ageing, or a response to certain chemicals in soaps and detergents.

5

CHILDREN'S FEET

A child's foot is not simply a scaled-down version of an adult's foot, but is different in several ways. For a start, the shape of a child's foot is different to that of an adult, as its widest point is across the toes, while in the adult it is widest across the metatarso-phalangeal joints. Also in the young child the feet will invariably look flat because the long-arch area is filled with a fatty pad of tissue which will remain until the child is actively walking.

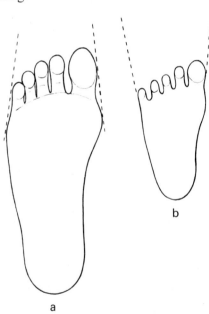

Differences between the foot shape of an adult and an infant.

The skeleton of the child's foot is also very different to that of the adult. When a child is born the bones in the foot are not fully developed; in fact some have not even appeared by the time the child is walking. The cuneiform bones appear during the child's first three years and the navicular, which is the last to appear, arrives in the third or fourth year. The bones that do appear in the new-born baby's foot will be mainly cartilage (gristle), which is soft and pliable, very unlike the bone in the adult's foot. Bone gradually replaces the cartilage as growth continues (a process known as ossification), but it is not until approximately 18 years of age that a young person's bones will have stopped growing.

The fact that the shape of a young child's foot is maintained by pliable cartilage rather than hard bone means that it can be easily malformed and compressed without causing discomfort

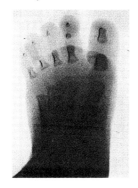

Six months

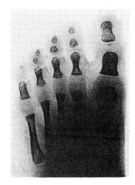

Two years

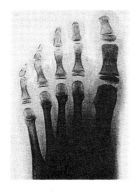

Eight years

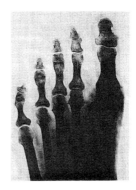

Adulthood

Development of the feet.

to its young owner. It is for this reason that great care must be taken in the fit and style of children's shoes – subjects looked at in depth in Chapter 9.

During the child's development the shape of the bones will also alter slightly so that the position of the foot, knee and hip in relation to each other will change.

THE CHILD'S GAIT

Most children between the ages of 12 and 18 months will be walking. They should not be encouraged to walk before they are ready and equipment which is meant to stimulate early walking is of dubious value (see page 17).

To begin with the child will walk with their feet wide apart, with a waddling gait. The normal heel-to-toe pattern of foot contact with the ground does not develop until the child is two or three years of age; instead they will use the foot as a single unit, which they pick up and put down at each step.

BOWLEGS AND KNOCK-KNEES

Bowlegs is a common occurrence in the new-born child and is considered to be within the normal development of a child until the age of two. Unless bowlegs are linked with a disease, such as rickets or other rare conditions which affect the growing part of the leg bones, then the bowlegs will normally correct themselves. During the early stages of walking a child with bowlegs will often have a flat (pronated) foot and will walk with an intoeing gait (pigeon-toed).

After the age of two it is normal for the legs to develop knock-knees which will be at their maximum at about the age of four, after which they will improve and correct themselves by the age of six. The foot will also be pronated (flat) during this stage.

FLAT FEET

Excessive pronation or flat feet is probably the commonest problem seen in the feet of young children, and can be associated with leg or foot misalignments or be part of normal development. Generally it is not painful, neither does it usually interfere with the normal activities of a lively child. A common complaint from parents whose child has this problem is the breakdown of the side of the shoe and excessive wear on the sole and heel of the shoe. The wearing of an insole to reduce the pronation usually reduces this damage to the shoe.

However, in some children it does cause discomfort and there is also a possibility that, although the condition is symptom-free, it may be the cause of many foot complaints which develop in later life. Various devices can be provided by the chiropodist or doctor which are placed into the shoe and act either on the heel, to control its movement, or on the foot generally. These devices, which are usually made of light-weight plastics, have to be made specifically for an individual child and should not be a mass-produced item taken off the shelf.

INTOEING AND OUT-TOEING

The intoeing and out-toeing of the foot during walking in the young child is not necessarily viewed as being abnormal and therefore requiring treatment. An intoeing gait is seen as a natural development in some toddlers, associated with the bowing of their legs.

The reasons for intoeing and out-toeing, although different, are both related in the main to leg and body actions during walking and to a lesser extent to any foot problems. The position and shape of the bones in the lower limb change during a child's development and this has an important influence on the foot's position during walking. The muscles in the thigh will also have an effect on the actions of the leg and the position of the foot during walking.

Although many cases of intoeing will certainly correct themselves during childhood as the bones in the lower limb rotate into their allotted positions, some will not. It is always advisable therefore, when worried by a marked intoeing or out-toeing, especially in a child over the age of seven, to seek professional advice.

NAIL PROBLEMS

Many of the toenail problems seen in the very young child will improve as the child gets older.

Curly nails
These can curl over the top of the toe and almost cut into the skin. They should be cut in the normal manner and should straighten themselves out by the age of two or three.

Thickened nails
Some children are born with a thickened toenail, the nail affected often being the one on the big toe. The chiropodist can reduce its thickness without causing any discomfort by using an electric drill, and this will have to be repeated two or three times a year to keep the nail looking normal.

Some cases do not improve as the child grows, and will produce a thickened nail that in adult life might need a more radical treatment.

Ingrowing toenails
This condition is not common in young children but is very common in the adolescent and young adult – see Chapter 4 for more details.

TOE PROBLEMS

Most children are born with perfectly-formed feet, but a small number will have minor toe problems. These will often take the form of two toes overlapping or one toe burrowing underneath another. Many chiropodists feel that with proper management these toes can be straightened and can be put back into a normal position. Before commencing any course of treatment, however, the shoes and socks should be checked for fit (see Chapter 9); a shoe that is too tight will hold a toe in its abnormal position and reduce the chances of achieving any correction.

The chiropodist may take a silicone rubber device that fits around the affected toes to hold them in a better position. The silicone starts as a soft putty or a runny paste and a catalyst is added to it which sets it into a firm rubber while it is being moulded onto the foot. The device, when finished, is fitted onto the toes and can be removed and replaced when washing or at bedtime. It also has the benefit of being washable, durable and non-allergenic, so it should not cause any damage or irritation to a child's skin.

An alternative, especially in the very young child who cannot be reasoned with, is the use of adhesive strapping which is used to reposition the toes. This normally requires replacing on a daily basis by a parent who must be trained by the chiropodist in the correct manner of application. If incorrectly applied the strapping could cause damage to delicate skin. This technique using adhesive strapping is likely to take several weeks or months, and can cause a skin reaction in some cases.

There is an old adage that it takes one month for each year of a child's life to produce correction in a mispositioned toe. However, once the child reaches early puberty, the chances of successful correction by strapping or silicone devices diminish.

BUNIONS

The movement of the big toe towards the outer border of the foot can be seen in young children in their fourth and fifth years. By the age of 18, over half of the female population will have a measurable amount of hallux valgus or bunion (see pages 31–4). The type of foot and its functioning during the normal walking cycle, plus the footwear and its suitability, all contribute to this sideways movement of the big toe.

Treatment using toe-straightening devices, strapping and exercises are generally disappointing once the toe has moved more than 15 degrees from its line with the first metatarsal bone. If the main underlying problem is one of foot imbalance an orthosis to fit in the shoe to improve the foot's function may prevent further deformity. However, if the deformity continues to progress it may be necessary in adult life to have surgical correction of the problem. More details about hallux valgus can be found in Chapter 3.

HEEL PAIN

In children between the ages of nine and 13 pain can occur in the heel, often bad enough to cause the child to limp. The problem is at the growing part of the heel bone where the rear part of it is pulled away from the main body of the bone.

This condition is known medically as Sever's disease and will usually settle down on its own, but the chiropodist may be able to help by providing a soft heel pad which fits into the shoe and raises the heel.

HEEL BUMP

In some adolescents a small bony lump develops at the back of the heel near the area where the Achilles tendon is inserted. Because of its prominence the back of the heel is likely to be rubbed by the shoe, producing pain and sometimes a bursa which can become red and swollen. This area is also very susceptible to chilblain formation during the winter months.

During the acute phase, when the area is painful and inflamed, the chiropodist may apply protective padding. It may be possible to break down the stiffener at the back of the shoe by hammering the leather. Another remedy is to raise the heel within the shoe with a heel pad which alters the position of the bony lump in relation to the back of the shoe. Surgery to remove the bony lump may be necessary in very troublesome cases.

PAIN IN CHILDREN'S FEET

There are two other areas in the foot, apart from the heel, which can suffer with problems often referred to as growing pains.

The high point of the inner long arch is where the navicular bone is situated and pain can be felt in this area in a condition known as Kohler's disease. The child affected is usually between four and 10 years of age, and it causes them to limp. The condition is thought to be caused by local pressure which reduces the blood supply to the growing area of the bone and is known as osteochondrosis of the navicular bone. Treatment is usually aimed at resting the area, and makes use of soft splinting with adhesive felt and strappings. It will take several months for the condition to clear and will need some support during this period.

A similar condition, in which the growing part of the second metatarsal bone is interrupted, causes pain near the ball of the foot in the adolescent foot. This condition is known as Freiberg's infraction and can be treated by padding on the sole of the foot which relieves pressure on the painful second metatarso-phalangeal joint area. An insole may be necessary to improve the foot's function during the condition's healing stages. Non-treatment is liable to lead to arthritic changes to the joint in later life.

SKIN

The formation of hard skin or corns on a child's foot is obviously a sign of a problem, usually caused by the shoe rubbing because it is a poor fit or a bad style. If a properly-fitted shoe does not lead to an improvement in the hard skin then the advice of the chiropodist should be sought, before any long-term damage occurs.

Juvenile plantar dermatosis
This condition affects the skin on the sole of the forefoot and especially the under-surface of the big toe, although it can extend to the top (the dorsal surface) of the toes. The skin will have a shiny, glazed appearance and will be peeling and scaly with, occasionally, some shallow splits in the skin. The cause of the problem is thought to be linked with sweat production, and is usually associated with non-absorbent socks or tights and shoes which are non-permeable, such as those with plastic or rubber uppers.

Treatment requires a change in footwear so that cotton or wool socks/tights are worn, and shoes should have leather uppers; if possible, sandals should be worn. An absorbent insole, made of leather fibreboard, inside the shoe is also helpful, but it must be replaced at regular intervals.

ATHLETE'S FOOT

This condition is seen more commonly in the older patient and is described in detail in Chapter 3, but it can affect all ages. It is especially important in the child's foot to clear the infection, and this will require the regular application of a fungicide cream. In the young child, when the medication is applied by the conscientious parent, then results are usually excellent. In the adolescent, when self-treatment is the norm, then the results are usually less spectacular.

VERRUCA PEDIS

The word verruca is Latin for wart. A verruca is caused by the same virus that produces warts on other parts of the body; it is a benign (mild, non-malignant) tumour of the skin and its difference in appearance when on the sole of the foot is due to pressure which flattens its outer surface. On the sole of the foot it may also become covered with a layer of hard skin which masks its true identity.

Cause
The virus is thought to be caught when the bare foot comes into contact with a surface that has been contaminated, such as the flooring of swimming baths, or sports changing rooms.

Comparison between corns and warts

	Corn	Wart
Age	Middle-aged/elderly	Children/young adults
Site	Over bony areas	Anywhere
Pain	Most painful on direct pressure	Most painful when squeezed
Duration	Takes months or years to develop	Takes days or weeks to develop
Appearance	Yellow hard centre	Tiny black spots within it

A virus cannot live very long outside a host so it must find entry into the skin through a minute break or injury, which in most people can be found on the sole of the foot. Once in the skin cell the virus will cause it to grow and divide to produce abnormal skin cells. This increase in cell division, plus the resulting problems with small blood vessels and nerves, causes a small tumour to form.

Consequences

The life history of a wart, once developed, will vary greatly. The body may produce antibodies against it and cause it to be shed, producing no more than a slight inconvenience to the patient. Surveys carried out show that approximately two-thirds of warts during a period of two years will disappear in this way.

The advice to most patients with a wart on their foot which is not painful and not increasing in size or number would be to leave it alone. It is a sensible idea to keep the wart covered with waterproof adhesive plaster (Sleek) when bathing or using public changing areas. Also because the infection can be transferred to other parts of the body, picking at the wart should be avoided and the towel that is used to dry the affected area should not be used elsewhere.

The possession of a wart on the foot should not interfere with a child's attendance for swimming lessons. The wart is of little consequence compared to the importance of being able to swim. If required it is possible to purchase thin rubber socks which slip over the feet (Brit Marine Guard Socks), and these should reduce the chance of infecting others whilst attending public baths, etc.

Treatment

If it is decided that treatment is necessary, then the chiropodist is usually the person best trained to diagnose and treat warts on the feet. However, you ought to remember that, while there are many treatments for the common wart, this does imply that no one treatment can provide a 100 per cent cure-rate. Some treatments are quicker and cleaner than others, but the suitability of any treatment will depend largely on the patient's general health, the site of the verruca, its size, its duration and what other treatments, if any, have been tried. You must also remember that most wart treatments aim at destroying the wart tissue and the virus contained within it, and this will inevitably cause the patient some discomfort during certain stages of treatment.

One problem with the treatment of a wart is that, during the process of treating it, tissue breakdown occurs in which the wart liquefies and produces a small ulcer or blister and perhaps some discharge. This does not mean that the wart is septic but is likely to mean that treatment has been successful; it is usually quite normal and of little consequence, but may worry the patient if not fully explained.

Chemical treatments

Various ointments and lotions can be used to treat warts. Most are strong caustics which can burn or damage the skin, so must always be used with caution. They must be applied in a controlled manner to avoid causing any damage to the healthy skin which surrounds the wart. Additionally, the warty tissue that is affected by the chemicals must be carefully removed before any more is applied. It is for these reasons that self-treatment using preparations containing caustics such as salicylic acid are usually unsuccessful.

Treatment using these preparations will usually take several weeks and will require the patient to keep the foot dry and the dressing in place between applications. Some lotions, such as glutaraldehyde and formalin, can be applied by the patient at home, although the results are slow compared to most other treatments. Thuja, which is a homeopathic remedy, can also be applied daily by the patient in its tincture form, but this also will be a slow treatment.

Freezing

This is known medically as cryotherapy and is used to lower the temperature of the wart to a level at which the cells die. The dead cells will liquefy into a blister, which is usually shed after a period of weeks, leaving the skin clear and unscarred.

The treatment produces some discomfort at its time of application, but in most other respects it is more convenient to the patient than the repeated application of ointments or lotions.

Electrosurgery

This method, sometimes known as fulguration or electrodesiccation, involves an electric current being used to dry out and cauterise (burn) the wart tissue. Before using this method a local anaesthetic is needed to reduce the discomfort which otherwise would be felt during treatment.

Curettage

The wart can be scooped out of the skin using a small spoon-shaped instrument. A local anaesthetic will be required before curetting, but the skin requires no stitches afterwards, the area healing quickly providing it is kept clean.

Occlusion

The strict and continuous use of a waterproof adhesive plaster over the wart can cause, after a few weeks, so much waterlogging to the area that the wart falls out or peels out attached to the plaster. However, to keep an area of the foot covered all the time, especially for children, can be very difficult, but if the plaster is left off for an hour or two the area will dry out and the treatment must be started again.

6

THE ELDERLY FOOT

As we get older our feet, like many other parts of our body, are liable to cause some problems. One of the reasons for this is the natural ageing process which affects the body's tissues such as the skin, joints, blood vessels, nerves and the fibro-fatty tissue under the skin.

The ageing of the skin is best illustrated by pinching a little loose skin up from the back of the hand and then releasing it. In the young person the elastic tissue in the skin will cause it to return to normal instantly. However, the older we get the slower the return, the poor recoil being linked to the reduction in the amount of elastic tissue present. Nourishment to the skin is also likely to be affected as we age, making the skin drier, thinner and in some cases devoid of any hair growth. These factors all contribute to the fact that the skin on the foot of the elderly is less tough and not such an effective protection barrier as in the young.

The blood supply in the foot is likely to be less efficient than in the young person due to the changes that can take place in the walls of the arteries. In addition, those people whose mobility is impaired will find that the pumping action of the calf muscle (see page 75) is reduced and the circulation becomes sluggish.

Poor circulation and fragile skin can lead to ulcers and poor healing, especially if aggravated by minor degrees of pressure. The protective layer of fibro-fatty padding over the areas of the foot which are most susceptible to stress reduces with age, leaving the metatarso-phalangeal joints without their efficient shock absorber. The result of this is that the skin on the foot is more likely to produce corns over these bony areas.

Professional help with the care of the elderly foot is particularly needed as problems with eyesight, coupled with arthritic hips and knees, make it increasingly difficult for the sufferer to reach and attend to their own feet. Arthritic joints within the foot also alter the way in which the person walks, making some joints more liable to overload in an effort to compensate for the inefficiency of others.

And finally, quite apart from the ageing process itself, the feet can be affected by many medical conditions associated with ageing, some of which may show themselves first in the feet. Some of the more common conditions are discussed in some detail below.

DIABETES

This condition is one of the most important because of its possible effects on the feet.

Diabetes produces an imbalance of sugar in the bloodstream which in turn can produce problems in different parts of the body such as the eyes, kidneys, nerves and blood vessels. If diabetes develops in a young person they are likely to be insulin-dependent and will therefore require injections of insulin daily to control their condition. If, however, the condition first appears in middle or later life it can often be controlled by diet or pills. It is believed that the better the diabetic patient controls their diabetes then the less serious will be the problems that arise in the blood vessels and other organs.

The two main areas which will affect the feet and lower limbs in the diabetic will be those involving the blood vessels and the peripheral nerves.

Vascular complications

The blood vessels which carry blood to the leg and foot can become reduced in diameter, so reducing the amount of blood circulating. Without a good and adequate supply of blood, the valuable nutrients, oxygen and the white blood cells which provide our defence against infection will be in short supply. The skin of the foot will respond by appearing poorly nourished – dry, shiny and hairless. The lack of oxygen will make the foot appear discoloured, often taking on a reddish-blue (cyanotic) colour. The reduced blood supply will also make the feet more susceptible to infections as the important white blood cells will be in smaller numbers compared to someone with a normal circulation.

It is even possible in some cases for the blood vessels to become blocked by a clot of blood. This is seen sometimes in the small arteries of the toes and if the obstruction causes a complete blockage the area of skin and tissue nourished by the blood vessels will start to suffer quite quickly. The area will eventually produce a darkened patch which is a localised area of dead tissue and termed gangrene. It is important that an area of gangrene is kept dry, clean and free of infection. If the circulation should improve, this area of dead tissue may simply be shed, but if the obstruction remains, the area may extend and require a surgeon's intervention.

Another possible complication for the diabetic patient with circulation problems is the appearance of ulcers on the foot. This is a more common problem than gangrene and is likely to have a successful outcome if treated by the chiropodist early enough. The most common site for a foot ulcer will be on those areas of the foot which are subject to damage from pressure and friction. The top of the toes, over enlarged bunion joints and under the metatarsal heads are all areas which are often affected. The ulcer starts in the deep tissues but is often uncovered when a chiropodist is treating the callous overlying a corn. This layer of callous or dead skin must be carefully removed to allow any discharge to escape and assist the edges of the wound to meet and heal. This removal usually causes the patient no discomfort.

Local relief can be provided by applying sponge or felt padding around the affected tissues. This helps to alleviate unwanted pressure falling on the area and speeds up recovery. In severe cases, general rest, which may mean total bed rest, is required until healing takes place.

If the ulcer is infected an antiseptic on a sterile gauze dressing is required. The chiropodist will often incorporate this dressing with the protective pad mentioned above. The chiropodist will also want to liaise with your doctor or consultant if he feels that antibiotic cover is required, or if he needs information about your diabetic control. The chiropodist, of course, is not the only member of the health care team involved in diabetic ulcer management. The nursing staff in the hospital and in the community will also be involved in treating some ulcers either independently or in conjunction with the chiropodist.

Ulcers can take many weeks to heal completely, and will cause the patient a good deal of inconvenience and worry. Prevention is a better alternative and good foot care should reduce the likelihood of any problems.

Neurological complications

The nerve supply to the foot can also be affected in the diabetic patient, producing areas of numbness over part or all of the foot. If an area is not sensitive to pain, damage can occur without the person realising it, and on the foot this can lead to ulceration. The damage can occur simply from a stone in the shoe, the seam of a sock rubbing or a drawing pin passing through a thin-soled shoe. These events in a normal foot will produce pain and therefore a reaction on the part of the individual – either they will slip off their shoe and remove the irritant or walk in a different way until able to deal with the problem. However, the diabetic's first indication of a problem might be when they examine their foot at the end of the day. Failure to keep a careful eye on the condition of their feet, or failure to ask others who have better sight to check for them, can mean that minor problems rapidly lead to more serious ones.

All diabetic patients would benefit from a foot examination by a qualified chiropodist, especially when first diagnosed. A diabetic who is well stabilised, with no nerve or vascular problems, should be able to care for his or her own feet without professional help, but regular care for those with nerve or vascular problems is likely to be essential if debilitating foot problems are to be prevented. For this reason most modern hospital diabetic clinics have a chiropodist as one of the health team.

FOOT CARE CHECKLIST FOR DIABETICS

Regular inspection

Check your feet regularly – at least once a day – to detect the early stages of blisters, swellings and any other minor damage to the skin. If you suffer with poor eyesight try to enlist the help of someone to check your feet for you.

Care of wounds

Cover any open sore with a clean, if possible sterile, dressing until the area heals. If the wound is not improving then consult your doctor or chiropodist immediately.

Self-treatment
Never use corn plasters or paints on your feet as they usually contain an acid which can damage the skin and other tissues of the diabetic patient. Never cut corns or callous yourself nor allow a friend to do it for you. Never cut down the sides of your toenails, and never probe down the sides or cuticle with a sharp instrument.

Footwear
Avoid wearing footwear which constricts or rubs on parts of your foot, especially the toes. A good shoe should not need to be 'broken in'.

Hosiery
Check your hosiery as a hole in a sock or a badly positioned seam in a pair of tights could cause skin damage.

Avoid anything that restricts the circulation in your legs or feet such as garters and home-made elastic bands for keeping up stockings and socks. Never use lambswool wrapped around a toe as this can seriously restrict the blood supply.

Bare feet
Avoid walking about bare foot to minimise any damage that could be caused by pins and other sharp objects. Even a dog's hair can penetrate the hard skin on the sole of the foot and if not removed will produce a small septic spot.

Heat and cold
Avoid extremes of temperature on your feet. Take special care with baths to ensure that the temperature does not exceed 43°C. Use a bath thermometer rather than relying on the sensitivity of your hands. Likewise be careful with uncovered hot water bottles and sitting too close to the fire. Chilled feet can produce chilblains which, in people with poor circulation, can lead to ulcers.

Seeking advice
Any corns, callous or toenail problems should be treated by a chiropodist. Also seek advice immediately if you notice:

- Any colour change in your leg or foot
- Any swelling or throbbing in your foot
- Any discharge from a break in the skin or from under a toenail or corn

POOR CIRCULATION

There are other conditions apart from diabetes which can affect the blood vessels and produce poor circulation in the legs and feet. Arteriosclerosis (hardening of the arteries), atheroma (the deposit of greasy material in the lining of the arteries) and Buerger's disease (narrowing of the arteries and veins, especially in the legs) can all lead to a reduced blood supply to the foot.

If the circulation to the leg is reduced the muscles in the calf become short of oxygen and a cramp-like pain occurs in the back of the leg. This pain can be bad enough to stop the sufferer from walking and the leg has to be rested for a few minutes before walking can commence again. This symptom of poor circulation in the lower limb is known medically as intermittent claudication (on and off limping) and is an indication that the foot requires special care.

Raynaud's disease

This is a condition that affects the arteries in the fingers and toes. In the normal individual, cold will cause the small blood vessels in the fingers and toes to close down temporarily in order to conserve heat, and then to open up fully when returned to a warmer environment. If someone suffers from Raynaud's disease then the return of the normal blood supply is delayed. The fingers go noticeably white when first reacting to the cold and later, as they return to normal, they go through a period when they are coloured blue and then bright red, at which stage they are usually painful.

When Raynaud's disease occurs in young women without any other cause it will often improve or disappear as they grow older. When occurring in older people it may be associated with other signs of poor circulation.

In some people the shut-off of the blood vessels causes problems with nourishment to the tissues, especially in the toes, causing them to become shortened and tapered in appearance.

CHILBLAINS

One consequence of poor circulation in the legs and feet may be chilblains, especially over those parts of the foot subject to pressure.

A chilblain is an area of inflammation where the skin has been damaged by cold. It seems to affect the young and old more than those aged in between, and the most common sites are the toes, under the metatarsal heads, over the bunion joint, and at the back of the heel.

When an area is first affected by the cold it will often look slightly purple, will feel cold and may itch or tingle. The next stage, when the foot becomes warm, is a more painful one, with intense itching, and the area becomes red, swollen and hot. If this itchy stage is prolonged the scratching by the sufferer, coupled with the swelling in the tissues, can cause the chilblain to break and ulcerate.

If you are a chilblain sufferer then your main aim should be to prevent the start of chilblains by taking precautions in the autumn months before the very cold weather arrives.

Preventative steps

Socks and tights should be warm and insulating, using materials such as wool or the new thermal insulating materials which are now becoming so readily available. Keeping your legs warm will help retain the heat in the blood as it travels to warm up the feet; therefore the wearing of trousers by females and 'long johns' by males will keep the limbs insulated and will result in the feet staying warmer.

Shoes must not be a tight fit. Boots are usually a sensible idea, especially those with a fleecy lining, providing that they are fitted well. The benefit of the fleecy lining is dependent on air being trapped between the layers of fleece and thereby acting as an insulator; if the fleece is compressed it contains little air and will not therefore provide adequate insulation and thus little benefit to the wearer. And the thicker the sole of the shoe the better, normally, will be its insulating properties.

Avoid extremes of temperature. Do not warm cold feet by placing them directly in front of the fire, placing them directly on a hot water bottle or soaking them in hot water. When you come indoors let your feet warm up gradually by keeping your outside footwear on until your feet are back to a normal temperature. Wet feet will be affected by cold more than dry feet, so ensure that they are dried as soon as possible after they are soaked by a winter shower.

Try to avoid sitting or standing still in one position for any length of time, as exercise, especially of the calf muscles, is important in aiding the circulation to and from your feet. The chairbound patient may find this difficult to achieve and may need assistance in raising their legs or in the provision of a gentle massage to tone up the sluggish circulation.

Treatment

Once the chilblain has formed, treatment can only help reduce the symptoms. In the early stages a mild stimulant such as non-staining iodine ointment massaged into the area may be beneficial. Chilblain ointments and creams bought from the chemist can be helpful during the itchy inflamed stage. Calamine lotion and witch hazel solution are old remedies which are also very effective during this irritating stage.

If the chilblain breaks down then an antiseptic and sterile dressing should be applied until the area can be seen by the chiropodist or doctor.

THE ARTHRITIC FOOT

The word arthritis is used as a term to describe a variety of symptoms and conditions which can affect joints.

Osteo-arthritis

Osteo-arthritis is a common source of pain in joints and is thought to be the result of years of wear and tear on the joint. The joint affected becomes less mobile because the slippery cartilage between the joint wears away so that bone grates directly on bone. The condition also produces a change in the shape of the bones so that surfaces that were once rounded become flat and no longer able to move smoothly over one another. Additionally, the structures around the joint (the ligaments and tendons) will shorten and tighten if the space between the bones reduces, and this also contributes to the stiffness of the joint.

Osteo-arthritis can be found in many of the joints of the foot in patients in their middle and later life. A common joint affected is the metatarso-phalangeal joint of the big toe; this is known as hallux rigidus or hallux limitus, and is described fully in Chapter 3. The lesser toes are also commonly affected, with the inter-phalangeal joints becoming fixed and the patient unable to straighten their toes. The joints in the mid-foot area can be affected too, and will produce pain in the long arch area.

No permanent cure can be found for osteo-arthritis, so most treatment will be aimed at reducing pain and improving mobility. In the acute stage, when it is painful, rest and ice packs may be useful. The rest to the area can sometimes be achieved by splinting with padding to restrict movement until the condition improves.

In the long term, however, gentle manipulation of the affected joints in order to improve their function, plus the use of heat in the form of wax foot baths or ultrasound, may be beneficial.

Rheumatoid arthritis

Rheumatoid arthritis is a more extensive problem than osteo-arthritis as it can affect many tissues and structures, including joints, skin, blood vessels and nerves. It starts earlier than osteo-arthritis, the patient often being in their thirties or forties.

Within the joint, inflammation causes damage to the joint lining and cartilage whilst the structures holding the joint together are also damaged. This means that the inside of the joint becomes very painful and easily distorted from its normal position. This can be seen clearly in the hand, where the fingers drift sideways towards the little finger.

In the foot, pain is often felt first over the metatarsal region, and in time the toes will follow the pattern of the fingers and move sideways towards the outer (lateral) border of the foot. The toes also become clawed and fixed so that the foot requires a shoe with much greater depth in the toe box than normal. This position of the toes will result in the fatty pad under the metatarsal heads moving forward, leaving these bones no longer protected from pressure. This will be likely to make the already sensitive metatarso-phalangeal joints even more painful and it is often necessary for the chiropodist to replace this fatty padding with adhesive cushioning material or cushioning insoles for the shoes.

The arthritis will also often affect the rear of the foot and the ankle, leading to a low-arched rigid foot which is mechanically very inefficient. The fixed bony deformities will often lead to hard skin and corns forming over the most prominent joints. Because of the patient's fragile skin and possible problems with nerves and blood vessels, these areas can easily break down, causing an ulcer. Careful treatment is therefore needed to keep these areas clear of infection and to provide protection so that damage does not continue. In some instances, if surgical footwear or shop-bought shoes cannot provide the comfort needed, the chiropodist may have to produce a special shoe for the patient, using soft plastics that mould to the foot.

The foot of the person with rheumatoid arthritis may develop many varied problems and is likely to benefit greatly from the skilled treatment of the chiropodist. However, you will remember that it is important for all patients receiving medication from their doctor to inform the chiropodist of the name and dosage of the drugs; this is even more important in the case of rheumatoid arthritis because certain drugs such as steroids can produce problems with the rate of healing and might therefore influence the chiropodist's treatment.

Surgery, too, can be beneficial for those with severe foot problems as it is possible to remove the metatarsal heads, allowing the metatarso-phalangeal joints to be straightened, along with the toes. The cosmetic effect and the pain relief from a successful operation can often produce very satisfactory results.

Gout

Gout is a most painful disease, and is a form of arthritis in which small crystals of uric acid are formed inside a joint, producing a violent inflammatory reaction. The reason for the development of these crystals in the joint is because of a high level of uric acid in the body fluids, which may in turn be due to diet, alcohol or a family history of gout.

The sufferer is usually a male and the joint most commonly affected is the big toe joint (the first metatarso-phalangeal joint), although other joints such as the knee, ankle and the heel/arch area of the foot can be affected. In an acute case the joint begins to swell and after a few hours becomes red and painful. The area will soon become too tender to touch and even small movements or the pressure of bedclothes will be enough to produce excruciating pain. An acute attack usually settles in five to 10 days, with the joint returning to normal; however the same joint can flare up several times during the course of a year unless controlled by medication.

During an acute attack drugs such as Colchicine or one of the non-steroidal anti-inflammatory drugs are often prescribed by the doctor to control the pain and help terminate the attack. Different types of drugs such as allopurinol are given to the chronic sufferer on a regular daily basis and their purpose is to keep the blood uric acid level low.

The gout sufferer may also require advice regarding their eating and drinking habits. By losing weight, obese patients may also help reduce the high level of uric acid in their blood stream. Advice regarding footwear or a soft shoe insert may be beneficial, but otherwise the chiropodist has only a minor role to play in the treatment of the gout sufferer.

SWELLING

Swelling (oedema) of the foot and ankle can occur for many different medical reasons, related to conditions such as varicose veins, heart and kidney problems and pregnancy. It can also occur as a result of sitting in one position for a long time – obviously, merely due to the effect of gravity, fluid will collect around the lower leg. Furthermore, the muscles in the back of the leg normally help in the movement of fluids around the lower limb, but will be unable to function properly in the person who is wheelchair-bound or who is restricted to a plane or train seat for several hours.

If the reason for the swelling is not obviously linked with a local problem such as a sprained ankle or sitting for long periods, then it is advisable for the sufferer to visit their general practitioner. However, whatever the reason, the sufferer can help themselves during the day by resting with their legs raised, thus helping gravity aid the fluid return. And rather than using just a foot-stool it is better for the person actually to lie down on a bed or sofa. It is also usually best if shoes and tights/socks are put on first thing in the morning, before the fluid has had time to gravitate to the feet. Shoes can certainly be a problem later in the day if swelling occurs, so it is useful if the shoes have a lace or other fastening which can be adjusted to meet any increase in size.

7

WHAT IS A GOOD SHOE?

Shoes are one of our most important purchases. No other item of clothing has such a direct effect on the health of the body than shoes (although some doubt has been cast on the wisdom of tight jeans and trousers).

This chapter deals with the various aspects that will affect the fit of shoes. When you are looking for shoes with any of the qualities described the information needed can usually be found on the shoe box, in the trade catalogue (kept by any shop) or by asking an assistant. If the information is not available by one of these means then probably the shoes don't have the qualities you are looking for.

LASTS

Almost all shoes are made on a last. In some cases this last also forms part of the mould when soles are injected onto the shoes during the manufacturing process.

A last is normally made of plastic, sometimes metal or wood. Its purpose is to act as a mould so that the shoe can be made around it and retain this shape after manufacture. It is not a model of the foot that the shoe is expected to fit, but it is designed to give the shoe the internal dimensions which will accommodate the foot. This includes allowances for movement, growth (if appropriate) and fashion.

A good last is an essential base for a good shoe, especially as the fashion content of a last can have an important bearing on the fit of the shoes made on it. Some major manufacturers compile detailed surveys of feet so that last shapes can be produced which will accommodate the feet and, where appropriate, give the shoe the stylish look required. The last will also determine the alignment of the foot in the shoe and should be designed so that there is no pressure on either side of the foot that may affect gait.

Two other important aspects of a good last are heel pitch and toe spring. If the heel pitch is incorrect the shoes made on that last will unbalance the wearer during walking. Toe spring also assists walking; it gives the sole its curve from the flex line forwards so that the foot can rock forward when taking a step. The less flexible the sole the more 'spring' is required, the most obvious example being a wooden clog, which has to have a very high toe spring otherwise the wearer would be unable to walk.

DESIGN

The conception of a new shoe, i.e. the design stage, would seem an obvious place to consider its fitting properties. Unfortunately, particularly at the cheaper end of the market, this consideration is found wanting. In such cases last shapes are produced to achieve a 'look', with no thought given to the foot shape which has to be accommodated. Many girls' fashion shoes, particularly imports, are made on women's lasts which have been graded down to children's sizes with no adjustment made for the different, still developing, foot.

The upper design is as crucial as that of the last. Careful design will ensure that there are no seams over the prominences of the foot which would cause pressure or friction. Consideration should also be given to the flexing areas of the shoe, so that it coincides with the natural bending of the foot. This functional aspect of design is vitally important and major branded manufacturers will fit-test each new last and style on many pairs of feet, critically appraising every aspect of the shoe at several stages through the design and development process before bulk manufacture is sanctioned.

UPPER MATERIALS

Whoever said 'You can't make a silk purse out of a sow's ear' could well have been a shoemaker, for it is true to say that quality shoes with good fitting properties can only be made out of the best materials.

Leather

Without doubt the best shoe upper material available is leather. No other material, natural or man-made, has all of its qualities. It is remarkable to think that it retains these qualities when it is only a byproduct of either milk or meat production.

In order that a shoe should fit around the foot it is necessary to shape the upper around a mould, i.e. the last. This shaping is partially achieved by carefully cutting the various pieces of the upper so that when they are stitched together they resemble the last shape. At this stage the **plasticity** of the leather is then needed so that when the upper is pulled over the last it will mould itself to its shape. This shape is then fixed into the upper by a process known as 'heat setting'.

When the shoes are worn the **elasticity** of the leather allows it to give as the feet alter shape but it will then recover to its lasted shape. This elasticity ensures that the natural functions of the feet are not inhibited by the shoe. A further advantage of these properties is that the leather will mould slightly to the individual characteristics of the foot, customising the fit of the shoe to the wearer.

Leather has a very high tensile **strength** which enables it to withstand the thousands of flexing actions which occur each day when walking. However, this property does vary in different types of animal skins.

Permeability is probably leather's single biggest advantage over other upper materials. Leather has a unique fibre structure which allows water vapour, in the form of perspiration, to permeate to the atmosphere. This is vital as there is a large concentration of sweat glands on the feet – each foot exudes about an egg-cup full of sweat every day. Sweating helps to regulate the temperature of the feet and the ability of leather to disperse the sweat helps to maintain a healthy environment for the feet, even under adverse conditions.

Virtually any **surface characteristic**, be it colour or finish, can be applied to leather. These range from a natural finish, showing the grain of the leather, through embossed finishes, using heated plates or rollers, to patents which today are usually PVC or polyurethane coatings applied to the surface of the leather. This type of patent finish does prevent the perspiration of the foot from permeating right through the leather, but in most cases, except when the wearer sweats excessively, the leather is able to absorb the perspiration and dissipate it when the shoe is off the foot. If a foot problem associated with heavy perspiring is suspected it is best to avoid this type of finish as a precaution. The other common finish used is suede, which is normally the pile or nap of the flesh side of the hide, enhanced by buffing.

Finally, leather is particularly **easy to work and maintain**. It can be stuck, stitched, tacked, split or cut easily during manufacture because of its fibrous structure. It is also easily cared for during wear providing the correct polishes, cleaners and protectors are used.

The main type of leather used for shoes today is cowhide. Smaller quantities of calf, goat, kid or pigskin are still used, but the fashion for alligator, crocodile and snake-skin shoes is diminishing, largely because these animals are killed only for their skins and also as the intricate pattern can now be reproduced on cow skin or synthetic materials.

Coated fabric

This material consists of a woven, knitted or random-laid backer with a PVC (polyvinyl chloride) or polyurethane (PU) coating. It is cheaper than leather but has few of its properties. It is used mainly for fashion footwear, especially ladies' shoes. It has little elasticity so its ability to mould to a foot shape during wear is limited. If a coated fabric shoe is a little tight when you buy it, it is likely to remain so. On closed-in styles its impermeability can lead to heat and moisture build-up which may result in bacterial growth in the shoe in some cases.

Cotton and woollen fabrics

These are normally only used as lining materials or for slippers or beach shoes. Their strength is poor compared to leather but the natural fibres, which are woven or knitted, do allow water vapour to pass through. The shape retention is poor so shoes tend to lose their shape during wear.

Poromerics

This name is derived from two words, poro (that which breathes) and meric (an association of substances in compound), and the material represents man's best attempt at copying leather.

Unfortunately it falls far short of its target. In comparison, its permeability and shape retention properties are only moderate and its poor flex/crack resistance can lead to some wear problems. Its cost also means that there are few poromeric shoes easily available.

Rubber and PVC
Both of these materials, particularly the latter, are used for Wellington boots. Hard-wearing and waterproof, they are excellent for muddy or wet conditions but not recommended for long periods of wear as the inability to release the foot perspiration causes a heat and moisture build-up and an ideal environment for the growth of bacteria.

Nylon
This is used mainly in conjunction with suede for trainers. The nylon itself is impermeable but the suede panels and the air holes, usually found in the waist of the shoes, which allow air to be pumped in and out during wear, help to cool the feet and prevent a perspiration build-up. Poor-quality nylons tend to fray at stitch holes but the better-standard nylons are extremely strong.

SOLING MATERIALS

Scientific advances have resulted in a greater variety of soling materials, with better wear and comfort than earlier materials, and this has led directly to more comfortable shoes. Traditional soling materials are still used but, whereas leather has no equal as an upper material, it has been superseded as a soling material.

Leather
This was the original soling material traditionally used for welted shoes (see page 89). The substance of the sole can cause the shoe to be inflexible if insufficient toe spring is built in, and this may lead to heel-fit problems.

The leather tends to wear quickly on surfaces such as concrete and tarmac, and will therefore need to be repaired or replaced several times during the life of the upper. This needs to be done professionally to prevent the shoe becoming unbalanced. Tread patterns cannot be cut into the leather so care has to be taken on wet or smooth surfaces as the slip resistance is poor in these conditions.

Rubber

This is still a very popular soling material and is found in many forms.

Crepe rubber (natural latex coagulated and milled into sheets) is used for sandals and desert boots. Its flexibility is affected by temperature but it wears well.

Vulcanised rubber (crepe mixed with sulphur and moulded with heat) is usually produced in its microcellular form today to reduce its weight and increase its shock absorption. It does have a tendency to wear at the edges, which in severe cases can unbalance the shoe if it is not repaired.

Resin rubber is a solid rubber which can be cut very thinly and used to copy lightweight leather sole features, but with better wear. It is normally found on ladies' fashion footwear.

Thermoplastic rubber (TR), like microcellular rubber, is a 'blown' material. It has good grip properties, wears quite well and can be injected into units or directly onto the upper.

Polyvinyl chloride (PVC)

This is a solid plastic material which is very hard-wearing and flexible. Its only minor disadvantage is its weight. It is one of the most popular soling materials used today.

Polyurethane

This is a complex chemical cellular structure which is the best soling material available today. It can be moulded in either solid or microcellular form and is very light, tough and flexible.

SHOE CONSTRUCTION

There are several shoemaking techniques in common use today. Some are traditional, others have been developed to improve comfort and fit. The major constructions are detailed below. However, these constructions are by no means the only ones available today; some manufacturers have developed their own unique constructions, specifically designed to improve comfort and fit.

In-lasted

This is the most popular construction method in use today. An insole is temporarily attached to the bottom of a last and the upper is pulled over to the shape of the last and secured to the insole. The lasted edge of the upper is prepared and then a sole is either stuck or injected onto the shoe.

This method is used for all types of footwear, including sports footwear, and gives reasonable flexibility.

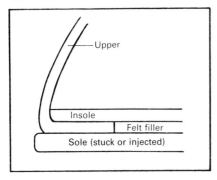

Inlasted shoe.

Veldtschoen or stitch-down

This is similar to the in-lasted construction except that the upper is turned outwards instead of under the last and is stuck to a wider insole, known as a 'runner'. The upper is then stitched to the runner and a sole is attached in the same way as the in-lasted construction.

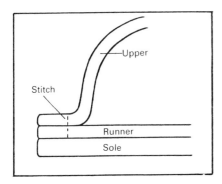

Veldtschoen or stitch-down shoe.

Slip or force lasted

The upper is stitched to a sock and, sometimes, a platform cover, the last is forced in and a platform stuck on. The platform cover, if used, is fitted over the platform and, whatever variation is used, a sole is then stuck or moulded on.

The platform is usually of a cellular material (PU foam) which is comfortable and shock-absorbing underfoot. The absence of an insole also gives a very flexible comfortable fit.

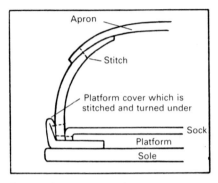

Slip or force lasted shoe.

String lasted

A string attached to the lasting edge pulls the upper over and around a light insole or sock in one operation. The sole is then injected on, in most cases, so that the string becomes embedded in the sole.

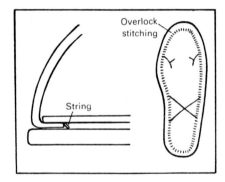

String lasted shoe.

This method is normally used for lightweight materials, and gives shoes good flexibility.

Moccasin
The upper passes under the foot and is completed by stitching in an apron. A last is forced into this 'bag' to give it shape.

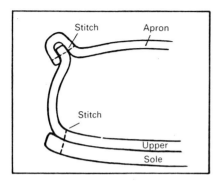

Moccasin shoe.

The construction does not necessitate an insole so is very light and flexible, and it has the added advantage of completely encompassing the foot in leather, giving added comfort and health properties.

Welted
This is a complicated traditional construction, normally used for men's formal footwear. The insole has a rib to which the upper and a welt are stitched. The welt is then flattened, the space between the rib filled, and the sole stitched on.

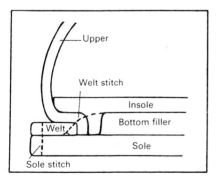

Welted shoe.

A welted shoe, although comparatively inflexible, is nevertheless a good quality shoe.

8

CORRECT SHOEFITTING

The 20th century has seen some of the most dramatic developments in nutrition and health care ever. People are now growing taller and heavier than ever before, and looking forward to an ever-increasing life expectancy. And this trend has obviously had a marked effect on the development of feet.

The average foot size of the population, both by age for children and of mature males and females, has increased tremendously. Many size ranges of mainstream footwear now include size 12, sometimes 13, for men and up to size 9 for women as the norm. No doubt the increasing number of people with feet beyond these sizes will result in even larger sizes being added to shoe ranges.

And foot girth (width) has also seen the same, if not a greater, increase occur over the same period. Average width fitting for children increased by almost a full fitting every 15 years during the middle of the century, and consequently manufacturers added extra fittings to their ranges to cope with this increase. Indeed today the leading children's manufacturers can offer as many as six width fittings. A similar trend has been seen in adults' footwear, where not only are wider shoes now required but a considerable number of wise adults also prefer comfortable non-damaging footwear to the excesses of fashion worn by many of their parents' generation.

This increase in foot girth has been accompanied by an equally dramatic change in the distribution of the foot volume, which is best illustrated by the pictures of typical children's lasts from the 1930s and 1980s seen opposite. The change in the foot profile, and the consequent change in the last profile, needed to accommodate this is self-evident in these pictures.

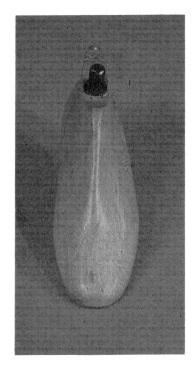 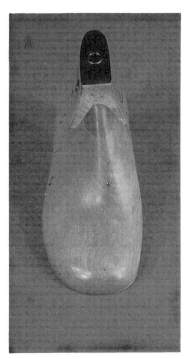

Child's last from the 1930s. Child's last from the 1980s.

One definite casualty of this evolution is the old wives' tale that gait problems could be corrected by swapping the shoes to opposite feet. Whilst in the 1930s this may not have created any extra pressure on the inner border of the foot (it probably had no effect on the gait either), today this practice is, quite rightly, labelled as barbaric.

THE IMPORTANCE OF WELL-FITTED SHOES

So just how important is the fit of our shoes? Ask a child, and they won't even be able to imagine the damage that a poor-fitting shoe can cause. Ask a teenager, and they'll tell you that corns and bunions come with your old age pension. Ask a young woman, and she will probably put fashion before fit. But ask a person who is suffering from foot problems as a result of poor-fitting shoes in earlier life, and the answer will be entirely different. Many wish for a pair of shoes that are comfortable, and long for the days when their feet allowed them to walk more than a few yards without pain.

Our feet are the foundation of our bodies. We require them to support us, move us around and allow us to participate in many different activities and sports, and, as our life expectancy increases, we expect them to do this for many more years than ever before. However, it is a sad fact that most foot problems are the result of abuse or neglect in earlier years. Perhaps if we felt the pain and inconvenience immediately we might give them more consideration.

And how many of these foot problems can we really blame on our shoes? Some people will tell you that their problems are hereditary – 'My mother had bunions and so did my grandmother so I shall have a bunion.' Studies of feet in races who have never worn shoes at all have shown instances of foot defects, and it is equally true that of all the many foot types that could be described as normal, there are some which are more prone to foot defects than others. So we know that foot types can be hereditary . . . but foot problems need not be.

The simple fact is that shoes are probably the major cause or aggravator of foot problems. Many of these problems are the result of little or no attention being paid to the fitting qualities of the shoes. Sadly, for some these problems are a result of their parents not ensuring their shoes fitted correctly when they were children. Whoever we are, whatever activity we undertake, great importance must be placed on the fit of our footwear. A little extra care taken in the selection of our shoes will protect our feet, and in return they will give a lifetime of pain-free service.

SHOE SIZING

The origin of shoe sizes is very ancient. If some historical accounts are to be believed, the English shoe size system, for example, can be traced back to the very beginnings of yards, feet and inches. At that time it was decreed that an inch would equal the length of three barley corns laid end to end. As this system became accepted, shoemakers, who would be commissioned to produce a pair of shoes for an individual, would lay barley corns alongside the feet to determine the length of the shoe that they would be required to make. The number of barley corns would determine the size of the shoe and it soon became accepted that a shoe size equalled one barley corn or one-third of an inch. And within the English size system this increment is still accepted today.

INCHES	CENTI METRES	PARIS POINTS	ENGLISH SIZES	AMERICAN Sizes Children's & Men's	AMERICAN Sizes Women's
3¹¹/₁₂					
4					
¹/₆	11	16	1	1	
¹/₃		17		2	
³/₆	12	18	2		
²/₃		19	3	3	
⁵/₆	13	20		4	
5			4		
	14	21	5	5	
	15	22		6	
		23	6		
6	16	24	7	7	
	17	25	8	8	
		26	9	9	
7	18	27		10	
	19	28	10		
		29	11	11	AMERICAN Sizes Women's
	20	30	12	12	
8	21	31	13	13	15
		32		1	25
	22	33	1		
	23	34	2	2	35
9		35	3	3	45
	24	36		4	55
	25	37	4		
		38	5	5	65
10	26	39	6	6	75
	27	40	7	7	85
		41		8	95
11	28	42	8		
	29	43	9	9	105
		44	10	10	115
	30	45		11	125
12		46	11		
	31	47	12	12	135
	32	48			

Comparison of shoe sizing systems.

The anomaly within this system, whereby the sizes end at 13 and continue again at size 1, can be traced back to the fact that in the early days of the sizing system only the very rich could afford shoes; even the children of the very rich did not wear shoes as such. For this reason size 1 was the first size worn by the children of the very rich as they reached adulthood and received their first proper pair of shoes.

It was not until the 1880s, when shoes were becoming more affordable, that the London shoemakers laid down a guideline of sizes against measurements in inches. The resulting system, based on an adult size 5 equalling 10 inches, can be seen in the comparison tables.

Other sizing systems in current use include the American sizing system which, as can be seen from the table, has a base of 3 and $11/12$th inches for children's size 0. Subsequently the American equivalent of an English shoe size will be approximately a half size bigger, i.e. English size 2 = American size $2\frac{1}{2}$. However, the American system changes its notation on adult sizes for ladies only. This becomes $1\frac{1}{2}$ sizes bigger instead of a half size, and is usually described differently, i.e. English ladies' 5 = American ladies' $6\frac{1}{2}$, described as 65. This somewhat confusing description may be easier to comprehend by referring to the comparison table.

The third and most widely used system is the Continental or Paris Point system. In the truest traditions of shoe sizing, this method, using centimetres, starts at zero and increases by $\frac{2}{3}$ of a centimetre for each increment, i.e. Continental size 1 = $\frac{2}{3}$ of a centimetre, Continental size 2 = $1\frac{1}{3}$ centimetres. No doubt those of you with decimalised brains will realise that there is no exact decimal equivalent of a third (without a recurring last digit) but, faced with the involved history of the English system, I suppose it is only fair that the Continental system has its own little anomaly. However, one advantage of this system is that its notation continues without repetition from 1 to 50 (and beyond) so that there is no confusion between adults' and children's sizes.

WIDTH SYSTEMS

As with the sizing system, so there are variations in the width system used. The use of the word 'width' itself (an almost universally accepted term) is somewhat confusing as it in fact refers to the girth fitting of the shoe at the widest part of the forepart. The equivalent position on the foot is at the base of the big toe, at the joint with the first metatarsal, passing around the foot over the joint of the little toe with the fifth metatarsal.

The width systems are indicated in both the American and English systems by either a letter or a number. Only a relatively small number of shoes made using the Continental system are made in width fittings or indeed have any fitting mark on them at all; those that do favour the number system or are simply marked narrow, medium and wide. Where a letter is used in the English size system there are differences between women's fittings and men's or children's fittings. Men's and children's fittings run from A (which equals 1 if the number system is used) to H (equals 8). A and B widths are no longer produced in bulk and the number of C and D to be found are limited as there are relatively few feet requiring these fittings today. Women's shoes almost always use letters and the American width system. (The American equivalent to the English letter system is two less, i.e. English E = American C.) Therefore, a girl moving from children's shoes to ladies' shoes would need to look for a different fitting letter (two less than her children's fitting) to find a suitable fit.

The sizing and width systems which I have described, although based on exact measurements, are guidelines only. No rules, regulations or standards exist which can force manufacturers to produce shoes to the exact dimensions laid down by the system. This is not necessarily a bad thing as the licence given to the last manufacturers and shoemakers enables them to produce shoes to fit all types of feet. However, as individuals it pays not to adopt the attitude that our feet will only fit into a certain size and fitting. Although we should know our approximate size, it may be necessary to try another size or fitting to achieve a better fit, especially where shoes have been made under one system and the sizes have been converted.

MEASURING DEVICES

Measuring devices are very useful tools for a shoe fitter. They are also a sign of a good shoe shop. A shop that has footgauges will probably have a stock of shoes in the sizes that the footgauge can measure and a choice of fittings in these sizes. However, a footgauge is only capable of giving an indication of the likely size and fitting required to fit those feet. This measuring exercise alone cannot guarantee that the shoe size indicated will fit and it is necessary to have the shoes checked by a trained shoe fitter.

There are many methods of measuring feet, ranging from a simple size stick to sophisticated electronic machines. Whatever method is used it is paramount that the device is used correctly by a trained operator, otherwise a false reading will be obtained.

Size stick

This is a simple length of wood or metal with a stop at one end and a sliding bar at the other. The size stick is positioned along the inner border of the foot with the stop touching the heel. The sliding bar is then gently pushed in to touch the longest toe. Along the body of the size stick a size scale is marked and these sizes can be read off when the sliding bar is in position.

With this device it is normal to add sizes to the reading given in order to select the correct shoe. This is normally 2–2½ sizes if the size stick is used with the customer seated.

Heel-to-ball device

This type of device measures length by calculation of the overall length of the foot from the distance measured between the heel and joint at the base of the great toe. Foot surveys have indicated that this distance is normally 70 per cent of the total foot length.

Manufacturers' footgauges

Most reputable shoe manufacturers have designed footgauges to be used when fitting their products. Therefore these footgauges should not be used when fitting shoes other than those made by that particular company.

Footgauges fall into two categories:

- Weight-bearing
- Non-weight-bearing

The weight-bearing footgauge measures the length and width of the foot whilst the customer is standing and the weight of the body has caused the foot to spread. From the foot length measured the footgauge displays the size likely to be required. At the same time the foot width at the toe joints is measured

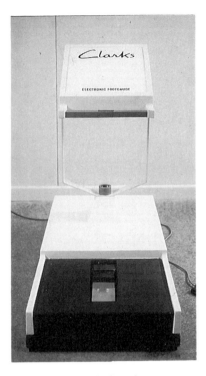

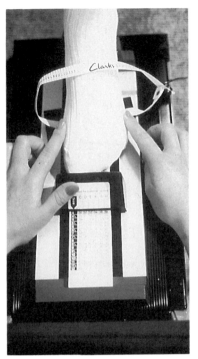

Electronic weight-bearing footgauge.

Non-weight-bearing footgauge for children and teenagers.

and the likely girth fitting required is calculated from this information and displayed.

The non-weight-bearing gauges measure the foot when its owner is seated; the foot is either held in the operator's hand or rests on a specially designed footstool. These gauges measure the length of the foot and add an allowance for weight bearing discovered from foot surveys. At the same time a tape is passed around the base of the toe joints and a girth reading is obtained.

Both groups of footgauges have advantages and disadvantages over each other, but providing they are used correctly they will give an experienced shoe fitter the likely shoe size and fitting required. Whatever method of measurement is used the most important factor is that the operator has been trained to use the footgauge correctly and to assess the fit of the shoes, subsequently selected, on the customer's feet.

9

FITTING CHILDREN'S FEET

Although it is important for shoes to fit at all ages, the stage when feet are most vulnerable is during childhood. During the 16–18 years that it takes for our feet to form fully, persistent pressure or too much room in shoes can lead to foot deformities.

If a child can reach their mid to late teens with undamaged feet they are also more capable of resisting, although they will be by no means immune from, the dubious fitting qualities of some of the fashion shoes worn by this age group.

EARLY STAGES

Shoes are not necessary for children until they are walking and need protection from the environment. There is certainly no evidence to suggest that putting a pair of shoes on a baby will make them walk sooner or better. Indeed, if a baby is learning learning to walk in the safe environment of the home, with carpets, adequate heating and no sharp or dangerous obstructions, they will probably master the art of walking quicker with the minimum of foot covering. Obviously the feet do need some sort of covering from the day we are born, but it is important to remember that these coverings can do as much harm as shoes, so careful attention is necessary.

Earliest consideration must be given to cot sheets and blankets which, if tucked in too tightly, can prevent the baby from kicking and moving. This exercise is vital to strengthen the muscles attached to the baby's developing skeletal system – the same muscles that will eventually allow the baby to stand and walk. All-in-one baby garments can also prevent this exercise if they are too short in the legs; this can easily happen as the baby rapidly grows or the garment shrinks in the wash. These garments need not be discarded at this stage, though, as the foot seams can be unpicked, hemmed and the garment worn with a pair of socks.

Pram shoes or knitted bootees, however pretty, are to be avoided unless they are replaced regularly. As feet grow so quickly in these early months this can prove costly. Most pram shoes are synthetic and therefore impermeable and their function can be better performed by good-fitting natural-fibre socks, at much less cost.

SOCKS

Socks must also fit well. Try to avoid buying wholly synthetic socks; although they wash better than wool or cotton, the tremendous stretch qualities of synthetics encourages manu-facturers to produce one sock size covering several shoe sizes. Invariably they are too big at the bottom end of the range and too small at the top end.

To check that socks fit correctly hold the foot part of the sock against the baby's foot. It should be as long as the baby's foot without being under tension. If it is the correct length the width-wise stretching of the sock to accommodate the volume of the foot will ensure a snug fit. Correct fit is essential as the tensile strength of sock materials, cotton and wool included, is greater than the resistance to pressure of the baby's cartilagi-nous bone structure. And check the seams of the socks thoroughly before purchase; if they are poorly finished and lumpy this will create pressure points on the foot when the socks are worn with shoes.

Finally, wholly synthetic socks create more friction inside the shoes than natural materials. This causes a heat build-up, excessive perspiring and a hot damp environment for the foot. It becomes increasingly difficult for even leather-uppered shoes to dissipate this extra moisture and creates an ideal breeding ground for bacteria.

WHERE TO BUY CHILDREN'S SHOES

When the time comes to purchase shoes, several factors must be considered. Children's feet are growing and developing

Logo of the Children's Foot Health Register.

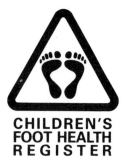

**CHILDREN'S
FOOT HEALTH
REGISTER**

constantly, and whilst this is happening it is vital that the feet have the necessary room in their shoes for this to occur. The immature nerve endings in the foot do not react so readily to pressure as those in adults' feet and consequently the child's feet can be squeezed and distorted without pain or discomfort.

To ensure that this does not happen a range of shoes in whole and half sizes, and available in several width fittings, is required. These shoes must be complemented by a trained shoe fitter who will measure both feet to obtain the likely size and fitting. Most importantly, the fitter will then check the selected shoes on the child's feet to ensure that every detail of fit is correct. Utilising their knowledge of feet and the fitting characteristics of the shoes, the fitter can make the necessary adjustments, if required, in width, length or shoe shape so that a good fit is achieved.

How, then, do you find a shop that can offer this service? Probably the best method is to consult a copy of the Children's Foot Health Register. The Register has the support of all the major bodies concerned with foot health in the United Kingdom, it is revised annually, and contains the names, addresses and telephone numbers of well over 1,000 shops who each year have given a signed undertaking to abide by the minimum standards of the Register. The promise is as follows:

- To stock children's shoes in whole and half length sizes from infants 3 to size 5½ for boys and for girls.
- To stock children's shoes in four width fittings.
- To employ trained staff to measure both feet.
- To ensure that shoes are carefully fitted by trained staff at the time of sale.

100

Copies of the Register are held by state registered chiropodists, health centres and some public libraries, or a copy can be obtained by writing to: Children's Foot Health Register, 84–88 Great Eastern Street, London EC2A 3ED, enclosing a 9 × 6 inch stamped addressed envelope.

Every shop included in the Register is under an obligation to indicate to the public, through prominent display of a current certificate of Children's Foot Health Register membership, that current Foot Health Register standards in stockholding and services are maintained in that specific shop.

Having found a suitable shop what sort of shoefitting training are the staff likely to have received? Most will have attended one or more training courses especially prepared by the shoe manufacturers, on which they will be instructed in the measurement and fitting of children's feet. Others may have attended their own company's training courses or those organised by the Society of Shoe Fitters. To add to these formal training courses, a competent shoe fitter needs good stock knowledge and – something for which there is no substitute – experience. The major manufacturers issue certificates to those who have attended their training courses, which will be on prominent display. They also issue badges, which the fitter will be wearing. If the shop staff are not wearing badges the simplest thing to do is to ask 'Are you a trained shoe fitter?'

MEASURING CHILDREN'S FEET

Without exception, the major manufacturers provide foot-gauges to assist in the fitting of their shoes. A good shoe fitter will always insist on measuring both feet, not just to obtain a shoe size and fitting but to have an opportunity to gain more knowledge of their characteristics. If the assistant just asks 'What size?' they are probably not a shoe fitter.

It is true that shoes can be fitted without a footgauge, but it is likely to be a time-consuming and frustrating exercise. Used by a trained person, a footgauge will, on the basis of two readings, length and width or girth, indicate a likely size and fitting. It cannot, however, predict the eventual fit of a pair of shoes on a multi-diametered movable object like the foot. This requires the trained skills and experience of the shoe fitter and a wide range of sizes and widths in shoes for them to select from.

WIDTH FITTINGS

Only about 40 per cent of children have an average foot width. That is to say, if a shoe is made in a single width fitting it will not fit, to the required standard, six out of ten children. To accommodate the range of foot widths found in over 96 per cent of the child population requires six different widths. The recognition of the increase in numbers of wider feet in this spectrum has prompted the leading children's shoe manufacturers to add the sixth fitting (H) to their ranges. The need for this wide range of fittings is probably best explained by describing the consequences for the child if only one width is available.

If a child has a wider-than-average foot a shoe of the correct length will be too narrow. To overcome this a longer shoe is required. This extra length results in the child flexing the shoe in the wrong place and extra creasing occurring at the toe, breaking down the stiffening which prevents the shoe collapsing onto the toes. In some cases the extra length is too acute for the child to cope with and can cause them to trip frequently, sometimes with serious consequences.

If the child has a narrower-than-average foot the single-fitting shoe of the correct size will be too wide. If the child continues to wear that shoe they will resort to 'clawing' the toes in an attempt to keep the shoes stable on the foot. This clawing can then easily become a feature of the foot. Alternatively, in order to reduce the girth, a shorter shoe is necessary which will cramp the toes and encourage the onset of hammer toes and hallux valgus.

As can be easily understood from this explanation, the consequences for both wide and narrow feet in average shoes can be dire. Every shop on the Children's Foot Health Register will stock shoes in at least four fittings, probably from D (narrow) to G (wide). In many cases these shops also stock either C (extra narrow) or H (extra wide), or possibly both. This fitting coverage means that it is possible to match the correct length and width for over 96 per cent of children 'off the shelf'.

CHECKING THE FIT

The most important part of a shoe fitter's job is to determine that the shoes selected actually fit the child. The criteria is quite simple. The feet should be able to perform all their normal functions without restriction or interference from the shoes.

To establish that this is the case, the fitter must methodically check every aspect of the shoe on the foot. In virtually all cases these checks should be carried out whilst the child is standing in the pair of shoes (having only one shoe on unbalances the child and nullifies the check), with weight evenly distributed on both feet.

Length

A correctly-fitting child's shoe should have at least half an inch of space internally in front of the longest toe. This allows for growth, movement and the toe shape of the last. If the toe shape is more styled an even greater allowance should be made.

As with most of these checks, the fitter uses their fingers to feel for the toe and judge the space available. If the toe of the shoe is too hard, talcum powder, liberally sprinkled inside the shoe before it is securely fastened on the foot, will leave an impression of the foot in the shoe after walking. The space available can then easily be seen by taking the shoe off and looking inside at the amount of undisturbed talcum powder. In this case it is important to remember that the movement allowance (one-sixth of an inch) has been taken up by walking in the shoes. This method is also useful to check shoes at home, although it is recommended that a qualified shoe fitter confirms the check. Any reputable shoe shop will happily provide a free fitting-check on shoes which they have sold.

Width and depth

These two features need careful assessment in tandem. Although two different lasts of the same size and fitting may have almost identical volume, the distribution of that volume may mean that only one of the last shapes is suitable for the foot being fitted. Sufficient space has to be allowed for the foot to function and grow without being excessive and causing discomfort through heavy creasing.

These checks will serve to confirm to the shoe fitter whether the footgauge reading is correct or a slight adjustment is required. Once this has been determined there are still several important checks to make. Most of these concern the middle and back sections of the shoe. In the middle and back of the foot there are, respectively, fewer and (particularly in the rear section of the foot) more cube-shaped bones; with the aid of some sort of fastening, these parts of the feet can happily withstand a shoe being attached to them. This allows the smaller and more easily damaged bones in the forefoot to develop without being under pressure. Good fit in this area requires the back curve to match the curvature of the heel so that the maximum grip can be achieved. Excessive height or curvature will result in pressure on the Achilles tendon, which could lead to bursitis. Conversely, insufficient heel curve or a low back will result in a loss of grip.

The topline of the shoe assists in back-part fit and should 'clip' neatly into the foot. At the same time the cut of the topline should allow clearance of the ankle bone, particularly the outer, unless the topline itself is padded in some way.

The well-defined inside arch of the foot also requires the shoe to follow its contours; excess material or lack of shape can both create pressure points in this area.

As indicated earlier, the fastening has a vital role in the fit of the shoe. There are several suitable methods of fastening available – bars and buckles, laces and, more recently, Velcro. Whichever of these methods is chosen it will be perfectly acceptable provided it is effective when the shoes are fitted and remains effective throughout the life of the shoe. Buckles present the least problem, and later in this chapter some tips to gain maximum benefit from laces and Velcro are given.

As a last static check of the overall effectiveness of the back-part fit, the back of the shoes should be tugged firmly, with the child sitting, to ensure that there is only minimal or no movement of the shoe. Any significant movement will lead to the child 'clawing' their toes in an attempt to keep the shoes stable.

The final test involves the child walking in the shoes. Some children find this difficult with an 'audience', but it is vital as it helps to confirm many of the static tests and ensures that the child can cope with the shoes without their natural gait being affected.

A trained shoe fitter can, using the procedure I have detailed, decide on the suitability of shoes on a child's feet. More importantly, they will spot the small faults which would go unnoticed by the layman. The skill of the shoe fitter in maintaining a child's foot health is as important as the work of the dentist or doctor is in keeping the rest of the child's body healthy.

USEFUL TIPS

- Don't hand fitted shoes down from one child to another. The shoes will have moulded to the first child's foot shape, and this will almost certainly be different to the characteristics of another child's foot, even if they are a brother or sister.
- Almost 80 per cent of children's shoes are sold on a Saturday or during short peak-selling periods (back to school). Try to avoid these times if possible, as the pressure on the staff of waiting customers increases the chances of mistakes occurring.
- Shop early at 'back to school' periods. Because of the cost of holding stock in many different fittings, most shops work on a 'fill-up' basis. At very busy times this can reduce the choice in the shops until the replacement shoes arrive.
- If you buy fitted shoes make sure your child is allowed to wear them at school. There are still some schools who care more about the state of their floors than the health of their pupils' feet.
- Don't let children wear slippers or Wellingtons for long periods. Short periods will do no harm, but in particular check the length regularly during the life of the footwear.
- Similarly, trainers should only be worn for long periods if they fit. This need not discount trainers; for example, Clarks produce a range in width fittings, with leather uppers if required, for the dedicated trainer wearer.
- Clean Velcro fastenings regularly; carpet fluff, dust, etc., will otherwise inhibit its grip.
- When teaching children to tie laces, pass one end over and under the other twice before pulling tight. This will lock the lace while the child forms the bows and make a more effective fastening.

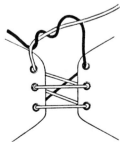

How to teach children to tie shoe laces.

10

FITTING ADULTS' FEET

Many people, even those who have had their shoes correctly fitted as children, pay little attention to the fit of their shoes on reaching adulthood. Even if this stage has been reached with perfectly-formed feet, continued abuse can cause severe and permanent problems. This does not mean that we have to restrict ourselves to 'fuddy-duddy' footwear at all times, but give more thought to the length of time we wear fashion shoes and consider the shoe's suitability for the activity undertaken.

For some people the decision about fit is very much their own. In many shops there are no facilities for measuring adult feet, or any advice forthcoming from the shop staff when choosing shoes. These types of shops should be avoided. It is true that, as adults, we are capable of making a shrewd judgment of the fit of shoes on our feet. However if this judgment is not based on the correct facts, then the wrong decision can easily be made. To minimise the chances, it is always wise to buy shoes from shops where your feet can be measured, the staff are trained in the skills of shoefitting and are knowledgeable about the stock in their shop.

Finding a suitable shop should not necessarily be too difficult. Almost certainly any shop that provides a children's fitting service will also provide a similar service for adults. Unlike children's shoes, however, the great variety of width fittings will probably not be available. Few adults' shoes are made in more than one width fitting, but often the range of styles available cover two or three width fittings. Some retailers stock several different brands of adults' shoes, in order to offer a greater variety of choice to the consumer.

As I have already suggested, it is wise to have both feet

measured, especially if you have not bought shoes from the shop before. This will enable the fitter to assist in the selection of a suitable size or style. In many cases this measurement will include checking the heel-to-ball length of the foot (see page 96). This measurement will determine the flex point of the foot in relation to its overall length. In most cases the heel-to-ball length will be approximately 70 per cent of the overall foot length and most shoes are designed so that the flex line of the shoe corresponds with this distance. In cases where this heel-to-ball length is different, an improved fit can be achieved by selecting a different size, as explained in the following examples:

If the foot length is size 5 and the heel-to-ball size is 6, this indicates a longer-than-average arch and correspondingly

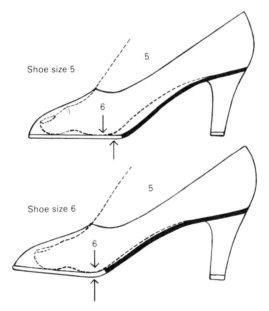

Shoe size 5

Shoe size 6

Fitting a longer than average arch.

shorter toes. In terms of length, a size 5 shoe would be long enough but, particularly in a heeled shoe, the arch would be under stress from the body weight and receive no support from the shoe. A size 6 shoe would give a better fit and more support, although there would be more length than required and a narrower shoe may be necessary to prevent the foot sliding forward.

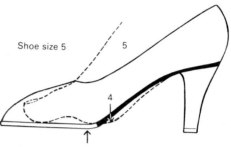

Fitting a shorter than average arch.

If the foot length is size 5 and the heel-to-ball length a size 4, this indicates a short arch and long toes. This can create a problem, particularly in shoes which are rigid behind the flex line. The foot obviously requires a shoe with sufficient length for the toes to operate, but if the ball position is behind the flex line it is difficult for the foot to function correctly and can force the shank through the sole bottom during wear. The shoes selected should therefore have greater flexibility; a moccasin for example, or, for women, an open-toe or a sling-back style, both with a lower heel if possible.

SELECTING AND CHECKING SHOES

When shoes have been selected it is necessary to check them as thoroughly as a child's shoe would be checked. Unlike children, who are continually outgrowing their shoes, an adult would expect to possess their shoes for a longer period, probably own several pairs at the same time and have bought each pair with one or more purposes in mind. These factors therefore have to be taken into consideration.

For a start, you must decide on the activities for which you intend to use the shoes. For example, if this is likely to involve a lot of walking or standing, then the stability of the shoes is essential; if they are to be worn for long periods, a leather upper will help to keep the foot cool and dry.

Basic fit and comfort

Are the basic fit and comfort of the shoe good enough? When checking shoes the following procedure should be followed.

- Always try on both shoes.
- Ask if the fit can be checked by the shop staff, and if so

ensure this is done whilst you are standing.
- If not, walk around the shop in the shoes, ensuring that your toes are not forced against the end of the shoe.
- Check that there is no pressure against the sides of the foot, especially at the toes.
- Ensure that there is sufficient depth in the forepart, but that it is not excessive – this would cause the upper to crease heavily on top of the foot.
- If there is a fastening make sure it is effective.
- Fastening or not, make sure the shoe does does not slip at the heel or cut in at the top of the heel curve.

Fashion and fit

And how will the fashion content of the shoes affect the fit? Although some men's styles are not totally blameless, it is in women's styles where the effects of fashion are most strongly felt.

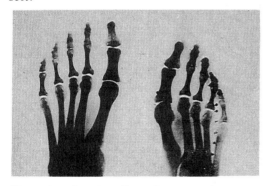

X-ray showing the effect of a court shoe.

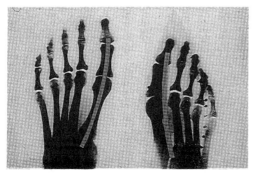

X-ray showing tendon bowstring effect.

Court shoes, in particular, which are non-adjustable, rely on the foot being held firmly either by sideways pressure or by the shortness of the forepart forcing the foot into the back of the shoe. Coupled with excessively pointed toe shapes, this has led to forefoot deformities such as hallux valgus and hammer toes for many women. In many cases the great toe is forced towards the other toes so far that the tendon which operates it becomes detached and instead of the toe being pulled upwards, as it should be, a 'bowstring' action occurs, pulling the toe even further over. High heels have contributed to these problems, as the body weight is forced onto the forefoot and the foot is held in such a position that the whole method of walking has to be adjusted.

It would be naive to think that these facts will stop women wearing court shoes, but it is possible to minimise the effects of these fashions with a little extra thought. Wear the highest heels and most pointed toes only when the occasion demands it. Wear more functional lower-heeled styles whenever possible. Don't wear courts or high-heeled styles at home; slippers or, better still, bare feet are best. With jeans or casual clothes wear trainers or other suitable flat shoes with a fastening.

USEFUL TIPS

- Feet get bigger as the day progresses so, to ensure court shoes don't get any tighter, buy them in the afternoon.
- If the shoes are loose in the morning or they have stretched, correct this by fitting a forepart insock to help hold the foot back. This can be removed, if necessary, as the feet get bigger during the day.
- Don't use heel grips to correct heel slip. This just forces the foot forward and jams the toes against the end of the shoe. Use a forepart insock instead.
- New leather-uppered shoes will become more supple and flexible in wear, but don't expect miracles. If they feel very tight or uncomfortable it's better to try an alternative.
- Synthetic shoes do not 'give' at all. If they are tight when you buy them, they will remain tight.
- Look after shoes. Shoe trees, cleaners and polish help to keep the shoes in good condition. And never force-dry wet shoes; allow them to dry at room temperature.

FITTING OLDER FEET

Old age brings with it problems such as poor circulation and brittle bones. The feet lose their resilience and the fatty tissue which has helped protect them in the past. Good footcare and shoefitting through childhood and young adulthood pay great dividends in later life, but even with good feet the need for correct shoefitting becomes more important as we grow older.

If the feet are generally undamaged then almost certainly good-fitting shoes have been worn, but two further factors must now be considered.

Firstly, if the feet are cold, opt for a style with a thicker sole or one with higher insulation properties, such as polyurethane. Thermal insoles can also be used, but always try the shoes with the insoles in position as the extra substance will otherwise make the shoes too tight.

Secondly, particularly for women, avoid high or unstable heels, as falls caused by these often lead to serious fractures. A style with a fastening will also assist in the stability of the shoes.

DAMAGED FEET

Unfortunately a large number of older feet are damaged in some way, more often than not as a result of poorly-fitting shoes. Wearing correctly-fitting shoes will not cure the problems, but it will certainly help to reduce pain and probably increase mobility.

There are several points to consider when selecting shoes for damaged feet. Firstly, it is essential to be measured, taking particular note of the heel-to-ball measurement. Over a period of time, if hammer toes and hallux valgus have developed, the feet will have shortened and it is quite likely that the shoes worn are smaller than required and are being flexed too far forward. If the correct heel-to-ball length is re-established then any movement left in the toe joints will not be restricted. Measuring will also indicate girth increase caused by hallux valgus and the associated bursa.

Secondly, most of the deformities will have developed in the forefoot, and to reduce the discomfort from shoes it is necessary to apply many of the principles of children's fitting,

111

i.e. the use of a fastening to hold the shoe securely onto the hindfoot so that the damaged forefoot can be relieved of much of the pressure put upon it. Damage to the toes is also likely to have increased their depth and the shoe must be able to accommodate them.

Lastly, many damaged feet will be swathed in a variety of padding or prescribed orthotics fitted by a state registered chiropodist. Particularly in the case of orthotics it is essential that the shoes are fitted with these in position so that their effectiveness does not destroy the fitting properties of the shoe or vice versa.

SHOEFITTING FOR DIABETICS

In addition to the advice concerning older and damaged feet, two further factors should be considered for diabetics.

Lack of blood supply and the loss of sensation in the feet means that diabetics have to take extra care with the fit of their shoes. This lack of blood supply is more serious than in cases of poor circulation brought on by age alone, and consequently a blister or ulcer caused by a badly-fitting shoe will take a considerably longer period to heal. The lack of sensation can also result in individuals not being aware of the damage as it is being caused.

- When buying shoes have them checked by a trained fitter and be sure to explain the problem to them.
- Have the shoes fitted with any prescribed pads or inserts in the shoes.
- Select shoes with soft leather uppers which will mould to the foot shape.
- Select a shoe with a flexible sole so that resistance to the foot's movement is at a minimum.
- Ensure that the foot is stable in the shoe and is held firmly by a suitable fastening.
- Check the interior of the shoes for poorly-finished seams or any other potential points of pressure.
- Each time the shoes are worn check inside for small stones, grit or other foreign bodies.
- Socks should not have any lumpy seams which will cause pressure points in the shoe.
- Socks should be changed regularly.

11

FOOTWEAR - RELATED ALLERGIES

A very small percentage, but nevertheless a significant number, of people suffer from allergic reactions to materials used in footwear. In many cases the actual allergen responsible for the problem is a chemical used in the production of the shoe component rather than the actual component itself. Because allergies are personal idiosyncrasies, an allergen-free shoe is impossible to produce, as without doubt someone somewhere would react to something used in the production of the shoe.

Stringent quality control is applied by the component and footwear manufacturers to ensure that no known dangerous substances are used. However, this fact will be of little comfort to those people who are allergic to the common substances used, to which the vast majority show no reaction. The range of materials available, and therefore the chemicals contained in them, is vast and can mean that isolation of the allergen is difficult. There are, however, a small number of well-known allergens, amongst whom the culprit can usually be found.

To assist those people who suspect they are suffering from an allergic reaction, the following advice and explanation may help bring relief from their suffering. If an allergy is suspected the first step must be to confirm this and identify the allergen. This requires consultation with a dermatologist, who will 'patch test' with the range of well-known allergens. If a positive reaction to one or more of the allergens is obtained it then becomes necessary to find footwear free of this chemical.

The well-known allergens, the footwear components in

113

which they are contained and some of the alternatives are detailed in this chapter, roughly in order of occurrence based on my own experience.

CHEMICALS USED IN RUBBER

- **Mercapto-benz-thiazole** (MBT)
- **Tetra-methyl-thiuram monosulphide** (TMT)
- **Diphenyl guanidine** (DPG)

Any one of these three chemicals will be used in the vulcanisation of rubber and identification of the rubber materials containing these chemicals is sometimes difficult. The soling material used may sometimes be stated on the shoe itself, on the shoe-box label or in the trade catalogue kept in the shop. Alternatively it will be necessary to contact the manufacturer.

Even if an allergy to only one of the chemicals is diagnosed, it is best to avoid vulcanised rubber altogether as, without reference to the rubber producer, the particular chemical used cannot be identified. Alternative soling materials are:

- Crepe and thermoplastic rubber (the chemicals in question are not used in the production of these materials)
- Polyvinyl chloride (PVC)
- Polyurethane (PU)
- Leather

CHEMICALS USED IN ADHESIVES

- **Para-tertiary-butyl-phenol formaldehyde** (PTBP, PTBPF)

This chemical is found in the polychloroprene (neoprene) group of adhesives. It is impossible for the untrained eye to detect this adhesive and its presence depends on the shoemaking process and whether each individual manufacturer chooses to use it or an alternative.

Major manufacturers are now using other bonding systems in preference to neoprene, thus giving a greater choice of styles for those who react to PTBP. The only sure way to avoid reaction is to contact the manufacturers and obtain a list of PTBP-free shoes.

- **Colophony** (rosin)

This chemical is found in adhesives, particularly EVA (ethyl-vinyl acetate) hot melts, which are much more frequently being used in shoe manufacture than in the past. As not all adhesives in the group contain this chemical it is difficult to identify the shoes to avoid, even for the manufacturer, who would have to consult their adhesive suppliers. And even if a reaction to this allergen is diagnosed there is now little alternative to this adhesive method. Fortunately the number of sufferers with this particular problem appears to be very small.

TANNING AGENTS

- **Potassium dichromate** (dichromate, chromate, chrome, chromium)

This chemical is used as a tanning agent in chrome and semi-chrome tanned leathers. The vast majority of leathers used in shoe manufacture are tanned by one of these methods and obtaining a pair of leather shoes not containing potassium dichromate is extremely difficult. Chrome-tanned leather fibres are also used in leatherboard. Although not used as frequently as it once was, it is necessary to ensure that the insole of the shoe is not of this material. Alternative materials are:

- Vegetable-tanned leathers – these are very difficult to find; you would need to contact manufacturers to determine whether they use leathers produced by this method.
- PVC or PU-coated fabrics, textile uppers (see Chapter 7).
- In the case of insoles, a cellulose or similar material.

DYES

It is extremely unlikely to find a material containing harmful dyestuffs. Diamines, which are known to cause more than just the odd allergic reaction, have been eradicated for this reason. Loose dyes are often blamed, when the culprit is often a sweat rash or something similar.

METALS

- **Nickel sulphate** (nickel)

This is occasionally found in the metallic components of the shoe (buckles, eyelets) which have been nickel-plated. Brass or the now commonly-used chromium-plated components provide a suitable alternative if a shoe without metal components cannot be found.

As styles change very quickly it is necessary for an allergy sufferer to have up-to-date information about footwear free of the particular allergen causing concern. Clarks Shoes produce lists of all their current styles free of the two most common group of allergens, i.e. rubber chemicals and PTBP resin, and can also provide advice on the other allergens mentioned in this chapter. A similar service may possibly be offered by other manufacturers.

12

THE FOOT AND SPORT

Since about the 1960s there has been a tremendous increase in the volume and range of different sporting activities undertaken by people of all ages. Most sports put stress on the lower limb, and the foot will often receive more than its fair share of damage. It is essential in almost all sports that the foot functions efficiently and is able to absorb both the forces coming up from the ground and the downward forces from the body.

The ability of the foot to pass from its position of pronation to supination smoothly and at the right stage during the cycle of walking and running is equally important. There are many different reasons why this normal process might not take place; they may be due to purely local foot problems or because of a problem higher up, in the leg, knee or hip.

A detailed biomechanical examination by the chiropodist must be made to identify the source of any problem. If the knee and hips are normal then the foot is likely to be the centre of the problem and must be carefully examined at rest with the patient relaxed on the examination couch, or by observing the dynamic foot and lower limb during its range of movements.

THE BIOMECHANICAL EXAMINATION

There may well be a biomechanical reason for many of the problems found in the sportsperson's foot and lower limb, and the chiropodist has a vital role to play in the diagnosis and treatment of many problems which up until recent years would have been untreatable or have required surgical intervention.

The foot is first placed so that the sub-tabloid joint is in its neutral position and then the forefoot is locked against the rearfoot. The chiropodist will then compare the position of the forefoot in relation to the rearfoot. If they are not in the same plane because one side of the forefoot is raised, then the foot is said to have a forefoot varus or forefoot valgus deformity, depending on its position.

Likewise the heel can be examined in relation to the leg; if it is turned inwards this is called rearfoot varus. Other variations from the normal range of movement are looked at and will include how much dorsiflexion can be achieved at the ankle joint and how much movement there is along the inner border and the outer border of the foot.

This is a simplistic description of part of the examination of the foot and must be supplemented by a detailed case history and by observing movements during walking and running where possible.

EXCESSIVE PRONATION

A problem caused by these minor variations from the normal is often an excessive amount of pronation, or the foot pronating when it should be supinating. This leads to the foot becoming unstable, producing abnormal stresses on the foot and possible reactions higher up in the knee, hip and back, which will in turn produce pain and functional problems.

The treatment of excessive pronation will often be centred around the production of a functional orthosis which is usually a lightweight plastic device which fits into the shoe and reduces the foot's necessity to compensate for a forefoot, rearfoot or leg problem. The device must be made accurately on a plaster of Paris case and is constructed with posting or wedges along its undersurface, which has the effect of bringing the ground to the foot rather than the foot having to twist itself abnormally to bring it into contact fully with the ground. The chiropodist will usually take the plaster of Paris impression of the foot, but the production of the orthosis may be undertaken by a specialist orthotic laboratory.

BLISTERS

A blister forms when a separation occurs between layers of skin cells; the space between these layers then fills with fluid. When blisters occur deeper, between the epidermis and dermis, then bleeding usually colours the fluid so a dark red/purple blood blister (haemotoma) results. Blisters may vary in size from tiny blisters (vesicles) no bigger than a pinhead in cases of athlete's foot to large blisters known as bullae which can occur in some inherited skin conditions.

The causes of blistering may be:

- Mechanical – known as friction blisters, usually associated with rubbing between the skin and the shoe, and commonly seen in sportspeople.
- Hot/cold – extremes of heat and cold can produce blisters; a typical example would be boiling water scalding the skin.
- Chemicals – the ingredients of adhesive plaster, iodine and some other chemicals can produce blistering in some sensitive individuals.
- Infection – a fungal infection can produce tiny blisters known as vesicles which will disappear when the fungal infection is successfully treated.
- Inherited skin conditions – a condition called epidermolysis bullosa can produce large blisters, which on the feet can be very disabling.

Treatment

The most common type of blister for most people will be the friction blister. This is best left intact where possible, allowing the fluid inside it to be reabsorbed by the body naturally.

If this process must be speeded up it is best not to remove the blister top but instead to pierce the blister with a sterile needle – two holes are usually needed so that the fluid can be gently squeezed out. The area should then be covered with a sterile dressing. Removing the blister top usually leads to a delay in the healing and a high chance of it becoming infected.

Prevention of blisters may be possible by following a few simple rules.

- If possible remove the reason for excessive friction on the part of the foot. Is the shoe badly designed or fitted?
- Wear two thin pairs of socks which allow the friction to

take place between the layers of socks.
- Use a light dusting of talcum powder in socks or tights.
- Protect likely blister sites by covering with a thin adhesive plaster.
- Prepare the feet several days before an event with surgical spirit or methylated spirit to harden the surface layers of the skin.

SHIN SPLINTS

This term is often used to describe any aching pain in the lower leg and may occur in most sports. The pain can occur in the front of the leg, along the outside border of the shin bone, in which case it is known as anterior shin splints, or it can occur in the muscles at the back of the leg, in the calf, and is then known as posterior shin splints.

The problem is usually one of muscle overuse which can cause pain within muscle compartments. Alternatively the fine attachments of the muscle to the bone can be pulled away, which also causes pain. There is usually a case history in which there has been a recent change in footwear or sports events, an increase in jumping, or a change to a harder running or playing surface. It is more likely to occur in the untrained or poorly-conditioned athlete at the start of the season rather than the well-prepared one.

Anterior shin splints
The pain usually occurs as a tightness after a period of prolonged exercise, but as the condition worsens it may be present during normal walking or even at rest. Feeling along the shin bone will produce some tenderness and in some cases small lumps may be felt.

The cause of the problem may be easily traced to a hard running surface. Running on concrete will cause a jarring effect as the heel comes into contact with the ground, and to reduce this trauma the muscles in the front of the leg are used more than usual, producing overuse pain. Other causes could include a tight muscle group in the calf forcing the muscles in the front of the leg to overwork, leading to muscle strain; or a foot that excessively pronates, and is therefore unstable, forcing the muscles in the leg to overwork in order to try and stabilise the foot.

Never try to run through the pain. During the acute stages ice packs can be applied to the muscle swelling to relieve the pain and inflammation. Running on hard surfaces should be avoided and soft cushioning insoles can be fitted into the shoes to provide shock absorbence. After the acute phase has settled gradual exercising of the anterior group of leg muscles can be encouraged. The chiropodist may be able to produce an orthosis to improve foot function if necessary and provide advice regarding methods of training until the problem is resolved.

Posterior shin splints

This produces symptoms in the posterior (calf) group of leg muscles and is usually associated with an excessively pronating foot which produces muscle strain. Treatment will be similar to anterior shin splints, with special emphasis on orthotic control to reduce the foot's pronation.

STRESS FRACTURE

The long bones such as the metatarsals in the foot and tibia and fibula in the lower leg are all prone to fracture if stressed enough. Although it is well understood that bones will break if struck hard enough or if one falls over, it is not as widely known that repeated minor stress such as marching or running can also cause bone fracture. The same effect can be seen if a rigid plastic or iron bar is continuously bent; it will fatigue at the bending point and eventually snap into two pieces.

The most common site of a stress fracture in the foot is the second or third metatarsal bone – often referred to as a march fracture. The pain may occur after a lot of walking, running or exercise and produce a swelling over the damaged metatarsal which can be felt on the top of the foot. The crack in the bone cannot be seen by X-ray during the early stages of the problem; indeed, it can only be detected by this method some two or three weeks after it has occurred.

The cause of the problem may be obviously linked with a change in training, footwear or running surface, but advice may be needed in case a foot imbalance is the underlying problem. Rest is essential to allow the hairline crack to heal, and this may take approximately six to eight weeks until normal training can recommence.

LIGAMENT STRAINS

The ligaments of the foot most commonly affected by sports injuries are the main ligaments of the ankle joint which are situated on both the inner and outer borders of the ankle.

The most common damage is to the ligaments on the outer (lateral) side of the foot – the lateral ankle ligaments. This sprain occurs when the foot is turned inwards towards the inner border of the leg. It occurs commonly in multi-directional sports but can also occur in running, especially on uneven surfaces, or even in the walker who trips off a pavement kerb.

The less common injury to the inner border of the ankle is known as a medial ankle ligament sprain. This can occur when the foot is forcibly everted – the sole of the foot turns outwards – and is seen in the very low-arched foot or in some contact sports such as football.

The degree of damage will vary from minor stress in the fibres of the ligament to a total rupture of the ligament, leaving the foot with an unstable ankle joint. However, even minor damage is likely to cause pain and swelling, even though this may only last for a few hours. More serious damage will be likely to produce persistent pain and swelling, normally accompanied by an area of bruising which, due to gravity, will form near the sole of the foot. Sometimes even a snap or tear is heard at the time of injury; this usually denotes a rupture or tear in the ligament and will have long-term consequences.

Treatment

As soon as possible after injury a cold compress such as a crepe bandage soaked in cold water should be wrapped around the ankle and ice packs should be placed over the bandage in the area of damage, with the leg if possible raised. The ice pack, compression bandage and elevation of the limb will all help reduce the swelling and pain that will otherwise result.

After these initial first aid measures a period wearing a crepe bandage or elastic anklet is often useful until pain and swelling has diminished. If the problem is slow to improve or is a recurring one, then your chiropodist or sports specialist may be helpful in providing advice on long-term management, using such apparatus as wobble boards which help exercise and re-establish the ligament's controlling function.

A more serious injury, where a partial or total tear of the ligament is suspected, should be seen in a hospital casualty department, who may wish to X-ray the joint. A complete tear may require a long period of rest with elastic strapping or with a plaster of Paris cast, but if this is not thought suitable surgery may be required.

TENDON PROBLEMS

Tendonitis (inflammation of a tendon) or tenosynovitis (inflammation of the covering of the tendon) can be caused by direct injury to the tendon or by its overuse or irritation. The direct injury might be a single sudden blow in a contact sport; the overuse may in fact be due to poor preparation and lack of stretching prior to exercise; and the irritation might be rubbing or pressure from a badly-fitted shoe.

The tendon of any muscle, if damaged, can become inflamed, leading to tendonitis in different areas of the foot, especially the inner and outer sides of the ankle and Achilles tendon. The Achilles tendon in particular may become painful at the back of the heel near its attachment to the heel bones, both during and after exercise. The inflammation may be bad enough to produce a visible swelling at the back of the heel and discomfort when just walking.

To treat tendonitis or tenosynovitis, rest and ice packs or cold compresses will initially be helpful, and these can be combined with a heel raise to relieve some of the strain on the tendon. As the pain reduces, gentle stretching exercises, combined with treatments such as ultrasound, may be prescribed by your chiropodist or sports specialist. During the healing stage training must be reduced, especially hill running, and only returned to a normal level slowly and gradually.

TENDO-ACHILLES RUPTURE

This powerful tendon can be ruptured during exercise, producing a sudden severe pain at the back of the heel and resulting in an immediate stop to the activity. It can occur in

123

an experienced athlete when the muscle is exhausted, but very often it is the response to too much exercise too soon in a person unaccustomed to strenuous activity. The best example is the poor dad who limps off the field during the fathers' race in the school sports.

The sufferer should attend the hospital casualty clinic where a plaster of Paris cast may be applied until healing can take place. In some cases surgery may be required to reattach the tendon if this is thought unlikely to occur naturally.

SPORTS FOOTWEAR

An increasing number of people, realising the benefits of regular exercise, are participating in sports which require specialist footwear. Because of this a considerable amount of research by manufacturers into the stresses and strains on feet, and the subsequent demands on the footwear during these sports, has been undertaken. As a result it is now possible to obtain a wide range of footwear designed for each individual sport or group of sports. Built into the footwear are many features to improve comfort, fit and support, and these will all enhance performance. Additionally a good-quality sports shoe will absorb most of the shock transmitted each time the foot strikes the ground, and is vital in reducing the number and seriousness of injuries that can result from strenuous activity. Cheap sports footwear invariably means cheap materials which have very limited durability and offer little shock absorption.

As a general rule a good brand name means a good shoe. In many cases the advantages of the shoe are given on an accompanying leaflet or swing tag – this can certainly be helpful when deciding what to buy. However, sports footwear is not generally made in fittings; therefore it may be necessary to try several brands before a suitable fit is achieved. Whichever brand is eventually purchased the following points should always be considered when buying and during use.

- Always try on the footwear with the appropriate socks. Many sportsmen or women wear two pairs of socks to reduce friction between the shoe and foot; others prefer one pair or even no socks at all. Provided the feet are not damaged there is no reason to change from your personal choice, but always ensure that new shoes are tried on as they will be used for the sport.

- Sports footwear has many pairs of eyelets and long laces to give the firmest possible attachment to the foot. It may take a little longer, but always fasten the shoes completely, as this critically affects the fit and comfort of the shoe. Never decide on suitability by just slipping the foot into the shoe and leaving the laces unfastened.

- When the shoes are fastened correctly and the weight is on the foot, ensure that there is at least one-sixth of an inch (4 mm) in front of the longest toe. During exercise a forward movement of the toes, even when the foot is firmly held by the laces, can be quite violent and cause blisters and abrasions if they continually rub against the end of the shoe.

- Shoes for indoor activities (squash, basketball, etc.) will have soles which give good grip on indoor surfaces. During wear the soles will pick up contaminants such as floor polish (from the changing rooms and corridors, if not from the court itself) and this will have an adverse effect on grip. To counteract this an occasional clean with a household cream cleanser scrubbed in with an old nail brush and rinsed off thoroughly with clean water will restore maximum grip.

- Outdoor sports shoes require considerable attention to retain maximum efficiency and increase their life. Clean thoroughly after use and dry out at room temperature but away from a direct source of heat. Stuff newspaper into the shoes so that they retain their shape and to prevent them drying out too quickly which, particularly for leather, will cause it to become hard and to crack.

- Leather should be treated with a polish or dubbin so that its suppleness is retained and water penetration is reduced when the shoes are next worn.

- Whether for indoor or outdoor use, sports shoes will absorb a considerable amount of perspiration during wear. Even if the footwear does not require cleaning after use, allow it to dry out at room temperature, otherwise the perspiration will literally rot the shoes.

13

SOLVING SHOEFITTING PROBLEMS

For the majority of people, buying good-fitting shoes presents no problems. All that is necessary is to visit shoe shops selling well-known brands of quality footwear with knowledgeable staff to offer advice. For others, however, buying shoes can present real problems. Happily there are many companies and bodies who can offer help. Information about them and the help available are contained in this chapter.

CHILDREN'S FOOT HEALTH REGISTER

This body is principally concerned with the prevention of foot problems rather than curing them. The Register lists over 1,000 shops offering a minimum stock coverage and a shoefitting service, covering the whole of the United Kingdom. It has the support of all of the major bodies concerned with foot health. Full details about the Register and its promises can be found in Chapter 9 (page 100); and its address can be found on page 136.

SOCIETY OF SHOE FITTERS

The Society exists to promote good foot health. Membership is individual and each member is required to demonstrate the required shoefitting skills and knowledge by completing a training course or by examination. Most of the members are

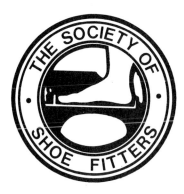
Logo of the Society of Shoe Fitters.

shoe retailers and can be consulted directly by members of the public in the shops where they work. Names, addresses and telephone numbers of members can be obtained from the Society (see page 136 for the address).

The extra knowledge of Society members enables them to help individuals with difficult fitting problems, and in many cases by having available a greater range of sizes and fittings than most shops. The range of services are listed below. It should be noted that the full range of services are not necessarily offered by every member.

- **Ladies' footwear**
  Large sizes over size 8 English
  Small sizes under size 3½ English
  Wide fittings E and over
  Narrow fittings B and double A
- **Men's footwear**
  Large sizes over size 11 English
  Small sizes under size 6 English
  Wide fitting F and over
  Narrow fitting under E
- **Children's footwear**
  Infant size 3 to boys' and girls' size 5½
  In half sizes
  In four width fittings
- **Others**
  Sports footwear
  Safety footwear
  Alterations and adjustments
  Catering to the handicapped

Orthopaedic footwear
Home visits
Odd size service
Made-to-measure service

Society members are also more than pleased to assist people who, although not suffering foot problems, just wish to take advantage of the best possible fitting service available.

BRITISH FOOTWEAR MANUFACTURERS' FEDERATION

Knowledge of the services available from its members enables the Federation to offer advice as to who best to contact when a special service is required. The Federation's address is on page 136.

DISABLED LIVING FOUNDATION

The Foundation is able to assist and advise people who do not consider themselves disabled, but who, nevertheless, find purchasing footwear a problem. This service arose from the research carried out by the Foundation and the information it has compiled in its superb efforts to improve all aspects of a disabled person's life.

The Foundation will provide, through the Footwear Adviser and at a very small cost, information on all types of footwear, manufacturers, shoe adaptations, footwear accessories, plus publications dealing with specific groups within the community and their footwear problems. The address of the Foundation can be found on page 136.

ODD SIZE SHOES

Names of companies offering this service can be obtained from the three organisations listed previously. Details of the service offered by Clarks Shoes Limited are as follows.

When individuals have large differences between their feet, either in size or width fitting, Clarks will take a special order to supply shoes in odd sizes and fittings in a limited range of styles. Delivery will normally take four or five working weeks, the shoes or sandals are specially made to order and as some styles have graded sole units this may require top piecing to balance the heel height. A surcharge of 25 per cent is made for shoes supplied under this scheme, to contribute towards the additional manufacturing costs. If top piecing is necessary, the surcharge is 30 per cent. If the odd shoes come from two size ranges, the price is averaged.

The service is available from Clarks fitting specialists, who will be able to provide further information about styles which are available under this scheme.

ORTHOPAEDIC ALTERATIONS

Most orthopaedic alterations will be made at the specific request of an orthopaedic surgeon or suchlike, and these will be referred to a suitably-qualified shoemaker known to the consultant. However, should one require shoe adjustments of the non-prescription type (caliper tubes, etc.), a list of qualified individuals can be obtained from the Disabled Living Foundation.

14

CHIROPODY IN BRITAIN

In 1960, state registration was introduced in the United Kingdom. Initially, it took in chiropodists who up to that time had not undertaken recognised training, as well as those who had, and state registration was given to them all. However, after that date only those who had trained at a recognised school of chiropody were granted registration.

Training involves a three-year, full-time course. Subjects studied include anatomy, physiology, microbiology (study of bacteria, viruses and other microscopic organisms), pathology (study of diseases), dermatology (study of the skin), medicine, surgery, and chiropody theory and practice. At the end of the course, students take the examinations of the Society of Chiropodists which allows them to use the letters MChS (Member of the Society of Chiropodists) after their name, or FChS (Fellow of the Society of Chiropodists) if they take further examinations. All those having passed the Society's examinations are then automatically eligible for state registration.

The state registered chiropodist is a specialist who provides a fully comprehensive foot health service for conditions affecting the foot and lower limbs. They have the right to treat patients without direction or referral from a doctor as they are responsible for their own diagnosis and treatment, including certain surgical treatments under local anaesthesia. The chiropodist must also be able to recognise those foot disorders which arise from general rather than local causes, and be able to treat them or refer them on to a specialist as appropriate.

Only state registered chiropodists are allowed to practise within the national health service. In private practice, however, there is no such protection and the public must choose between the registered and the large number who are ineligible for registration. Some such unregistered chiropodists will have undertaken postal courses, but as these courses are not recognised by the state, they cannot describe themselves as state registered chiropodists. And other unregistered chiropodists have no training or qualifications at all.

WHERE IS TREATMENT AVAILABLE?

Private practice
Most large towns will have at least one state registered chiropodist in private practice; by looking through the telephone directory such registered chiropodists should be easily recognised by the letters SRCh after their names. And remember, it is illegal to describe yourself as a state registered chiropodist unless you have undertaken the recognised three years' training.

National health service
Most hospitals, health centres and community clinics in the UK have a chiropodist who is in attendance either full-time or part-time.

Many health authorities give priority to certain groups of people who are then able to receive treatment free of charge. The normal groups are:

- Males over 65 years of age
- Females over 60 years of age
- School children and pre-school children
- Physically disabled
- Expectant mothers

The category which includes the disabled can be viewed in a broad sense to include medical problems such as diabetes and rheumatoid arthritis, or can be used in a very narrow sense to cover only those with severe physical disability.

If you are eligible for treatment then you can apply directly to the district chiropodist in your health authority or to your local health clinics. You may prefer to seek the advice of your GP or consultant, both of whom can also refer you to the health authority's chiropody service.

For those who are housebound a chiropodist may be able to make home visits, although not all health authorities undertake such domiciliary visits but instead provide ambulance or hospital car services to get patients to clinics.

Foot care assistant
In the UK health service an assistant to the state registered chiropodist has evolved who, under supervision, can undertake certain duties related to foot care. The extent to which this foot care assistant is involved in the treatment of the patient is likely to be small, but will vary throughout the country. The assistant is usually trained by the health service staff whilst in post.

Industry and commerce
Many of the larger companies such as food stores, department stores and manufacturing industries have a chiropodist who is a full-time member of the health care team or who visits on a sessional basis to treat the employees during their working day.

GLOSSARY

Abduct To move away from the midline of the body.

Achilles tendon The large tendon at the back of the leg attached to the heel bone.

Acute A condition having a rapid onset and a short and relatively severe course.

Adduct To move towards the midline of the body.

Allergen A substance or chemical to which an individual shows an adverse reaction.

Analgesic An agent which alleviates pain.

Anhidrosis Deficiency in sweating.

Anterior The front of a structure.

Apron The piece of shoe material on the top of the foot – usually in a moccasin.

Arthritis Inflammation of the joint.

Arthrodesis Surgical fixing of a joint to stop movement.

Arthroplasty Surgical intervention to produce a moveable joint.

Athlete's foot A fungus infection of the skin of the foot.

Back curve The shape of the back of a shoe.

Bilateral Both sides of a structure.

Blister A separation between layers of the skin which becomes filled with fluid.

Blown Term used to describe a microcellular soling material.

Bowlegs A condition where the ankles are together and the knees are apart.

Bromidrosis Sweating which produces a foul smell.

Bulla A large blister.

Bunion Inflammation and prominence of the first metatarso-phalangeal joint.

Bunionette Inflammation and prominence of the fifth metatarso-phalangeal joint.

Bursa A fluid-filled sack or cavity which is found in tissues where friction would otherwise develop. They may be normal or develop as a response to irritation.

Bursitis Inflammation of a bursa.

Calcaneum The heel bone.

Callous A thickening and overgrowth of the epidermal skin, usually as a response to pressure or friction.

Cartilage The smooth gristle-like tissue which lines those parts of the bone inside the joint which move over one another.

Cavus A highly-arched foot.

Chilblain Damage to the tissues caused by cold which produces pain, redness, swelling and itching, especially on the extremities such as the fingers, toes and ears.

Chiropodist Someone who specialises in the prevention and treatment of disorders of the foot.

Chronic A condition continuing over a long time or which tends to recur.

Club foot A gross deformity in which the foot is turned inwards and downwards.

Condyle A prominent portion of a bone.

Congenital A condition present at birth.

Corn A hard, cone-shaped thickening of the skin which results from pressure usually over a bony prominence.

Court shoe A relatively low-cut shoe with no method of adjustment, which slips on to the foot.

Cryosurgery Using extreme cold to destroy unwanted tissue.

Dislocation The displacement of the ends of the bones within a joint.

Distal The point furthest away from the centre of the body. The tips of the toes are the most distal part of the foot for example.

Dorsal The top surface of the foot.

Dorsiflexion The movement that takes place when the foot or part of the foot moves upwards towards the leg.

Embossed A finish applied to leather with heated plates.

Eversion A movement where the foot is turned outwards so that the sole is pointing away from the mid-line of the body.

Exostosis A benign bony outgrowth causing a spur or projection from the bone's surface.

Femur The thigh bone.

Fibula The smaller and outer bone of the lower leg.

Fissure A split in the skin.

Flex point The point at which the foot or shoe bends naturally.

Forefoot valgus The forefoot is turned out (everted) from the mid-line of the body in relationship to the heel.

Fracture A break in bone.

Gait The way we walk.

Genu varum Bow legs.

Girth In shoefitting terms, the girth normally refers to the *circumference* of the foot measured at the centre of the first and fifth metatarso-phalangeal joints.

Grain A leather finish which allows the natural characteristics of the leather to show through.

Haemotoma A blood blister.

Hallux The big toe.

Hallux rigidus A condition in which there is a reduction of movement in the big toe joint.

Hallux valgus A condition in which the big toe moves sideways towards the middle of the foot, and articulates abnormally. The metatarsal is then exposed, producing a prominence which is prone to pressure or friction.

Hammertoe   A deformity of a toe when it becomes buckled and fixed.

Heat setting   The fixing of the upper shape to the last contours by a combination of heat and moisture.

Heel grips   Self-adhesive pads which can be stuck in the back of the shoes.

Heel pitch   The vertical distance from the bottom of the heel curve of a last to the ground.

Heel-to-ball length   The distance measured along the inner border of the foot from a point at the back of the heel to the middle point of the first metatarso-phalangeal joint.

Hide   The skin of an animal, usually bovine, often used in shoe manufacture.

Hyperhidrosis   Excessive sweating.

Impermeability   The ability of a material to prevent perspiration or vapour passing through it.

Inflammation   The body's response to damage – the classic signs are redness, heat, swelling and pain.

Ingrowing toenail   A painful condition in which the toenail pierces the skin of the nail groove.

Insock   The piece of material used to cover the insole in a shoe. An additional insock may be used to improve the fit.

Insole   The 'foundation' of many shoe constructions. The insole is the same shape as the last bottom, and it is to this that the upper is attached.

Interphalangeal joints   The joints of the toes.

Inversion   A movement which causes the sole of the foot or part of the foot to turn inwards towards the mid-line of the body.

Involuted toenail   A condition in which the side of the toenail is excessively curved.

Ischaemia   Insufficient blood supply to the tissues.

Knock knees   A condition where the knees are together and the ankles are apart.

Last   The mould around which a shoe is made to give it its internal dimensions.

Lasting edge   The portion of a shoe upper attached to the insole during the making process.

Lateral   The side away from the mid-line of the body.

Ligaments   Fibrous tissue which connects bone to bone.

Longitudinal arch   The arch along the inner side of the foot –from the heel to the ball of the foot.

Matrix   The growing area of the nail.

Medial   The side towards the mid-line of the body.

Metatarsalgia   Pain in the area of the metatarsals.

Metatarsals   The five long bones connecting the rear part of the foot (tarsus) to the toes.

Metatarso-phalangeal joint   The joint between the head of the metatarsal and the base of the proximal phalanx.

Microcellular   Containing thousands of minute air pockets which reduce weight and increase shock absorption.

Morton's toe   Plantar digital neuritis, also known as Morton's metatarsalgia or neuroma.

Mycosis   Any condition caused by a fungus e.g. athlete's foot.

Non-weight-bearing footgauge   A footgauge which measures the foot whilst the customer is seated.

Oedema   Swelling.

Onychocryptosis   Ingrowing toenail.

Onychogryphosis   Thickening and distortion of the toenail.

Onychomycosis   Fungal infection of the toenail.

Orthosis   A device used to correct or stabilise the foot and so improve its function.

Paronychia   Inflammation of the nail and surrounding area.

Partial nail avulsion   Removal of a side section of a toenail.

Patch testing   A method of identifying an allergen by applying a small amount of the substance under a patch onto the skin.

Patella   The knee bone.

Patent   Normally a synthetic finish to leather or a synthetic to give a shiny durable surface.

Permeability   The ability of a material to allow perspiration or vapour to pass through, and thus to 'breathe' because of its fibrous structure.

Pes   The Latin for foot.

Pes cavus   A highly-arched foot.

Pes planus   A flat foot.

Phalanges   Bones of the toes or fingers.

Plantar digital neuritis   A pain in the cleft of the third and fourth toes. Also known as Morton's toe.

Plantar fascia   The fibrous band that is attached to the heel bone and the forefoot.

Plantar flexion   The movement which takes place when the foot or part of the foot moves downwards away from the front of the leg.

Plantar surface   The sole of the foot.

Pod   The Greek for foot (podos).

Podiatrist   A chiropodist who specialises in the surgical management of foot problems. Or the name given to chiropodists outside the UK, e.g. in Australia.

Posterior   The rear or back of a structure.

Pronation   The flattening of the foot to the ground involving three foot movements – dorsiflexion, eversion and abduction.

Proximal   A part which is situated nearest to the centre of the body, e.g. the knee is more proximal than the ankle.

Runner   The name used to describe the extended insole used in the veldtschoen or stitchdown construction.

Sensory Relating to sensation.

Septic Infected.

Sesamoids Small bones found in tendons, e.g. under the big toe joint are two sesamoid bones.

Shank A metal or wooden strip shaped to the profile of a last bottom to the rear of the flexline which will enable the shoe to maintain this shape on the foot.

Shin splints Pain and discomfort in the legs usually as a result of sporting overuse.

Shoe tree A shaped wooden or plastic block which helps keep shoes in good condition when off the foot.

Sprain A tear in a ligament.

Spur A bony projection or outgrowth, e.g. a calcaneal spur.

SRCh State Registered Chiropodist.

Stress fracture A break in a bone caused by overuse, also known as a march or fatigue fracture.

Subluxation A partial dislocation of a joint.

Subtalar joint The joint beneath the ankle between the talus and the calcaneum.

Sub-ungual Underneath the nail plate.

Supination The opposite movement to pronation which produces a more rigid arched foot. It involves three foot movements – plantar flexion, inversion and adduction.

Symptom Description given by the patient of their condition.

Systemic A condition affecting the whole body.

Talipes equinovarus Club foot.

Talus The highest bone in the foot situated between the leg bones and the heel bone.

Tendons Elastic tissue which connects muscles to bones.

Tendinitis Inflammation of a tendon or tendon covering.

Tenosynovitis Inflammation between tendon and tendon sheath.

Tibia The shin bone. The larger of the two bones of the lower leg.

Tinea pedis The medical term for athlete's foot.

Toe spring The distance from the tip of the toe of a shoe last at its base to the ground.

Total nail avulsion The removal of the whole nail plate.

Trauma Injury.

Ulcer An open sore.

Upper The top part of a shoe.

Valgus An abnormality in which the foot or part of the foot is angled away from the midline of the body.

Varus An abnormality in which the foot or part of the foot is angled towards the midline of the body.

Verruca The Latin for wart.

Weight-bearing footgauge A footgauge which measures the foot whilst the shoe customer is standing.

Width fitting The designation given to a shoe to indicate its internal volume – particularly at the toe joints (see **girth**).

USEFUL ADDRESSES

UNITED KINGDOM

Age Concern
Bernard Sunley House
60 Pitcairn Road
Mitcham
Surrey CR4 3LL
Tel: 01-640 5431
Fact sheets on the needs of the elderly including footcare.

Arthritis and Rheumatism Council
41 Eagle Street
London WC1R 4AR
Tel: 01-405 8572
Information sheets available.

British Diabetic Association
10 Queen Anne Street
London W1M 0BD
Tel: 01-323 1531
Fact sheets on footcare for diabetics.

British Footwear Manufacturers' Federation
Royalty House
72 Dean Street
London W1
Tel: 01-437 5573
Send stamped addressed envelope.

Children's Foot Health Register
84–88 Great Eastern Street
London EC2A 3ED
Tel: 01-739 2071
Include 9″ × 6″ stamped addressed envelope.

Disabled Living Foundation
380–384 Harrow Road
London W9 2HU
Tel: 01-289 6111
Information on footwear, hose and aids for the disabled.

Foot Health Council
84–88 Great Eastern Street
London EC2A 3ED

Health Education Authority
78 New Oxford Street
London WC1 1AH
Tel: 01-631 0930
Leaflets and resource lists about footcare.

Help the Aged
St James' Walk
London EC1R 0BE
Tel: 01-253 0253
Leaflets about footcare for the elderly.

National Consumer Council
18 Queen Anne's Gate
London SW1H 9AA
Tel: 01-222 9501
Information on footwear for children.

Office of Fair Trading
Field House
Room 310A
15–25 Bream's Buildings
London EC4 1PR
Or local Citizens' Advice Bureaux, Trading Standards or Consumer Protection Departments or Consumer Advice Centres for leaflets on the Code of Practice, covering the buying of shoes and repairs.

Royal Society for the Prevention of Accidents
Cannon House
The Priory Queensway
Birmingham B4 6BS
Publications on protection against foot injuries.

The Society of Chiropodists
53 Welbeck Street
London W1M 7HE
Tel: 01-486 3381
Leaflets on footcare and advice about chiropodists in private practice.

Society of Shoe Fitters
Farley Court
Farley Hill
Reading
Berkshire RG7 1TT
Tel: 0734 733931

Republic of Ireland

The Society of Chiropodists of Ireland
The Secretary
44 Annaville Park
Dundrum Road
Dublin 14

Australia

Australian Podiatry Council
Suite 26
456 St Kilda Road
Melbourne
Victoria 3004
Tel: (03) 266 8115

State Registration Boards

New South Wales
The Chiropodists' Registration Board
Mc Kell House
Rawson Place
Sydney
New South Wales 2000
Tel: (02) 217 6666

Queensland
The Podiatrists' Board of Queensland
9th Floor
280 Adelaide Street
Brisbane
Queensland 4000
Tel: (07) 227 7111

South Australia
The Chiropody Board of South Australia
c/o Mr L.J. Stewart
PO Box 62 Norwood
South Australia 5067
Tel: (08) 332 2477

Tasmania
The Podiatrists Registration Board
c/o Department of Health Services
Davey Street
Hobart
Tasmania 7000
Tel: (002) 30 8011

Victoria
The Chiropodists' Registration Board of Victoria
9th Floor
555 Collins Street
Melbourne
Victoria 3000
Tel: (03) 616 8059

Western Australia
The Podiatrists' Registration Board of Western
Australia
15 Rheola Street
West Perth
Western Australia 6005
Tel: (09) 481 0977

Austria
Member of FIP
Verband Osterreichischer Fusspfleger (VOF)
5030 Salzburg
Kaigasse 32
Tel: 83 2 92
President: Ms M. Schicho

Belgium
Member of FIP
Association Belge De Podologues (ABP)
Avenue Crokaert 97
1150 Bruxelles
Belgium
Tel: 02 770 50 86
President: Ms S. Charlier

Denmark
Member of FIP
Landsforenigen Af Stat. Fodterapeuter (L.as.F)
Bjelkees Alle 43
2200 Kobenhavn N
Denmark
Tel: 01 85 14 90
President: Ms B. Baunsgaard

Finland
Suomen Jalkojenhoitajain Liito R.Y. (SJHL)
Ludvigin Katu 7B.7
00130 Helsinki 13
President: Ms S.L. Reiman

France
Member of FIP
Fédération Nationale des Podologues (FNP)
163 Rue St-Honoré
75001 Paris
France
Tel: 4 260 62 45
President: Mr J.L. Emonet
NB In France a podologist has to be a French
national under their 1946 law, to practise.

Germany (West)
Member of FIP
Zentralverband der Fusspfleger Deutschlands (ZFD)
Urgingerstrasse 22
4130 Moers/Rhein
President: Mr K. Hamme

Italy
Member of FIP
Associazione Italiana Podologi (AIP)
Via Toscolona 713
00174 Roma
Italy
Tel: 39 6 768 973
President: Mr Mauro Montesi

Member of FIP
Associazione Nazionale Italiana Podologi (ANIP)
Via Ramazzini 3
20129 Milano
Italy
Tel: 272 597
President: Mr G. Zanetti

Netherlands
Nederlande Vereniging van Podotherapeuten
Postbus 32 58
5203 DG's – Hertogenbosch
Holland
Secretary: Mr M. Klitsie

New Zealand
The New Zealand Society of Podiatrists Incorporated
48 Witham Street
Island Bay
Wellington
New Zealand

Spain
Federation Espagnole des Podologues
C/San Bernado
74 Baso Derecha
28015 Madrid
President: Mr Julio Garcia Martinez

Sweden
Sveriges Fotterapeuters
Riksforbund
Regementsgatan 11
831 41 Osterund
Sweden

Switzerland
Member of FIP
Union des Associations Romandes des Pedicures
(UARP)
23 Rue du Grand Pré
1202 Genève
Switzerland
President: Ms P. Mota

Schweizerischer Podologen Verband (SPV)
Weisse Gasse 15
4002 Basel
President: Ms Heidi Quain

United States of America
The American Podiatric Medical Association
20 Chevy Chase Circle NW
Washington DC 20015
Tel: 202 537 4900
President: Mr K.J. Schwartz DPM

INDEX